Fertility Fuel

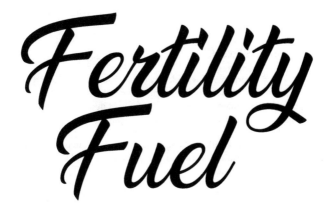

Fertility Fuel

Create Your Family Without Losing
Your Mind, Your Marriage, or Your Money

Susan G. Schiff, D.O.M.

NEW YORK

LONDON • NASHVILLE • MELBOURNE • VANCOUVER

Fertility Fuel

Create Your Family Without Losing Your Mind, Your Marriage, or Your Money

Published in New York, New York, by Morgan James Publishing in partnership with Difference Press. Morgan James is a trademark of Morgan James, LLC. www.MorganJamesPublishing.com

ISBN 9781642792584 paperback
ISBN 9781642792591 eBook
ISBN 9781642793178 audio
Library of Congress Control Number: 2018910617

Cover Design by:
Megan Dillon
megan@creativeninjadesigns.com

Interior Design by:
Chris Treccani
www.3dogcreative.net

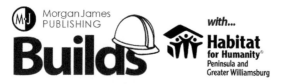

Morgan James is a proud partner of Habitat for Humanity Peninsula and Greater Williamsburg. Partners in building since 2006.

Get involved today! Visit
MorganJamesPublishing.com/giving-back

Dedication

This book is dedicated to my parents, JS and JS, who believed in me ... even when I took the convoluted, long, and wild road less traveled. My grandmother Bess, who always told me that she'd "put her money on me," and of course to my wife, Andrea, for being my co-conspirator in creating a full and adventurous life, and our son Tiger ... my constant teacher, unrelenting mirror, and my "Oliver."

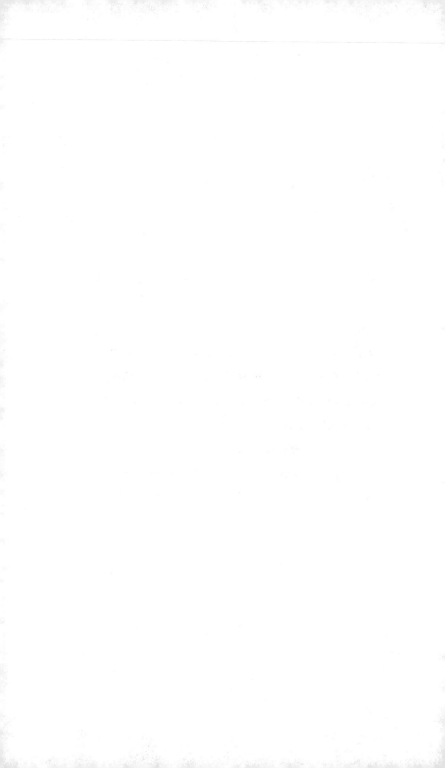

Table of Contents

An Appreciation

Dr. Susan Schiff has birthed Fertility Fuel through a long journey – personal, professional, and soulful. As we say in Chinese medical lingo, it came from her marrow. This is Susan's life, and her tremendous desire to help overcome the suffering you may presently be experiencing.

Anyone who has struggled with fertility is familiar with a desperate longing that few others know. Susan understands. She offers you not only hope, but many years of experience in this field. I met Susan many years ago, even before Tiger lit up her life. We've remained in the same group of fertility experts and friends ever since – sharing, learning, teaching, expanding, and growing together; and hopefully becoming wiser for it. And what unites us is the passion to heal. To offer a new way of approaching fertility that can change your life, too. Helping you to expand, grow, and become wiser on your journey toward parenthood. Who wouldn't want that?

Chinese medicine does not provide recipes. Life is too miraculously varied for that. Right ingredients do not end up turning into a baby. But right living can, while providing you with the fuel you need to propel you through this journey. There is no end point. I urge you to take one eye off the goal, and turn it inward. This is the most courageous journey you've embarked on, and the spark of new life is a by-product of that.

This is not merely a map. Dr. Schiff knows the territory, and she walks with you, sharing her wisdom, and very practical guidance step by step. She speaks directly, sharing stories of hope, fortitude, and the courage it takes to change the path you've been walking. Take a deep breath. Are you ready to take it in?

Randine Lewis, Ph. D., L.Ac., FABORM
Author of The Infertility Cure and The Way of The Fertile Soul

Foreword

You NEED to read Dr. Schiff's book and follow her advice if you want to maximize your odds of having another life come to you. Sure, there are dozens of acupuncture/fertility books and resources available, but none of them compares to the book you are now reading. Every acupuncture doctor brings something different to the table, but no one brings the breadth and depth of knowledge and experience to you the way that Dr. Susan Schiff can or will.

I spent 28 years of my life working my way through an educational system that would result in the realization of my dream to become Board Certified in Reproductive Endocrinology and Infertility. Having completed my Fellowship in Reproductive Medicine at the UCSD School of Medicine, I began practicing what I was taught and quickly realized that something very, very significant was missing in my training. My schooling showed me how to diagnose and treat fertility problems, but it ignored so many important aspects of who my patients really were: what were they thinking about their fertility problems, how were their challenges affecting their relationships with family members, friends, and work, and what was going on in their lives and within their bodies that might be contributing to the abnormalities I found on their blood tests but for which I had no good explanation?

After a short time in practice, I realized my Western Medicine-based educational perspective fell very flat. My search for answers as to why Western Medicine didn't "tick all of the boxes" for my patients led me to read and learn about Eastern Medicine practices. I opted to incorporate acupuncture into my patients' care as it was widely available and accessible to the majority of my patients. My practice paradigm soon led me to proffer an "East meets West" philosophy of practice.

After 17 years of helping fertility-challenged patients in New Jersey, I relocated to South Florida due to the better weather and the dire need for a fertility expert in Palm Beach County. As I had sent my NJ patients for acupuncture with improved pregnancy outcomes, I then needed to find a fertility acupuncturist in my new locale who can help accelerate my already above-average pregnancy rates.

Everyone I asked told me I *must* connect with Dr. Susan Schiff. I obtained her contact information, called her, and asked her to meet me so I could interview her and see if she was a good fit for my patients. Dr. Schiff and I jived in personalities and we mutually agreed to offer our patients the best of both worlds from our different medical perspectives. Soon thereafter we were invited to lecture to a group of Orthodox Jewish rabbis in Miami. That day was incredibly special because our lecture was well received but was also the day that Susan received a phone call stating that her baby (Tiger) was ready to be adopted!

Dr. Schiff and I have collaborated for the past 12 years. I have known scores of fertility acupuncturists during my career's three decades but have not met another practitioner who rivals her background, knowledge, techniques, and holistic healing approach. She focuses on *all* aspects of her patients' care, starting with the story of their birth, through the traumas they've encountered thereafter into adulthood, along with the balance (OK, mostly the imbalance) of their minds and bodies along the way. Like the innumerable patients I've sent to Dr. Susan, *you*, too, can benefit from her expertise by reading through this book and following her advice.

Much of what Dr. Schiff discusses herein relates to your lifestyle choices (Chapters Four and Five). You *are* what you eat. She is learned in our habits, food choices, activity levels, and nutritional supplements that can leave your body's soil sterile or can alternatively turn your soil into a nourishing host to best grow another life inside you for three quarters of a year. *Listen* to what she's trying to teach you. Be *open* to her words of advice and wisdom. Let her help till and enrich your soil. Her lessons in this book are invaluable.

Chapter Seven, "You Are Not Your Labs," highlights some of the reasons my Western Medicine training let me down. I was taught to check hormone levels and various other factors in your blood. I was told to count follicles on your ultrasound exams. I was supposed to check meaningless factors such as the clarity and stretchiness of your cervical mucus. My schooling said a man's sperm count had to be at least fifteen million. But these are just numbers on a piece of paper (OK, I'm showing my age, they're numbers on a computer monitor). All it takes to become pregnant, after all, is one good egg and one good sperm. And your age is a number, too.

Of course pregnancy success declines as a woman ages, but it does not necessarily mean you cannot conceive at an older age!

Try to stay the course, as discussed in Chapter Eight. If you do hang in there, you may be surprised and find you've crossed the finish line. Babies come to us in various ways such as pregnancy and adoption, and your life's path will bring you to something you were meant to achieve in the end. If you follow Dr. Schiff's advice, at the very most you'll find that child you've longed for, but at the very least you'll certainly find yourself healthier. And, as you've heard before, "If you don't have your health, you have nothing."

Wishing you the best in health and success!

Scott Roseff, MD, FACOG
IVFMD - Boca Raton, FL
www.IVFMD.com

Introduction

I am sure that you never thought you would be at this juncture in your life. Let's get real. Most women spend so much time, effort, and energy trying *not* to get pregnant. How can it even be possible that now that you *want* it to happen it's not? How many times have you semi freaked out when you forgot to take your birth control pill for a few days and thought that there might be a slim chance that you could be pregnant? Oh my God, not now. I'm just graduating high school. I just got accepted into law school. I just landed the promotion I've been working my whole life for. I just met this guy, I don't know if he's the one. It's so not fair. Yes, it is not fair.

I have met you. You are successful. You are smart and driven. Responsible. You're a good person. You are amazing. You set your mind on achieving something and you go all in. You're the author of your life. A doer. A go-getter. A driver. You have worked hard and it's mostly paid off. You *finally* met an amazing man that you want to spend the rest of your life with. Incredible to have finally met him! I know there were times when you thought that you might never meet him. Maybe you knew at first and maybe you didn't. It worked out and now you are ready. Let's do this. You stopped taking birth control. You have been trying month after month. You know it might take a few months, so you don't give it much thought. You start to notice that everywhere you go lately, everyone seems to be pregnant. You ignore it at first. Month after month, you are getting your period and it's starting to get to you. Maybe you should see your gynecologist. Maybe something is not right. You make an appointment. You're ready to take charge and get some answers. There has to be a reason. You're 36 and your doctor recommends you see a specialist. A reproductive endocrinologist. You're thinking that your doctor is being responsible and covering all the bases. You make an appointment with the specialist and your husband comes along. You both take off from work and are excited to go get some answers! The appointment is overwhelming. Your husband was shocked that both of you needed to be tested to assess your fertility prognosis. You both leave shocked, but resolute in doing whatever it takes – because doctors know best and we are good patients. It's now two years later and still no baby.

It's been a rough two years. All kinds of tests. You've been riding the roller coaster from your worst nightmare. The emotional infertility roller coaster that routinely engulfs you in sadness, frustration, anger, impatience, rage, shame, and grief. There are fleeting moments of "What if this is the month?" But mostly it's not fun. It's slowly eaten away at the joy and hope that you have created in your life.

By the time you read this, you might be exhausted. Emotionally, physically, and spiritually. The mainstream process of infertility *is* depleting. It's also very limited in its approach and you suspect that there are options.

My Invitation to You

I invite you to broaden your lens and look at the bigger picture around creating a life. Creating a family is probably the most important thing that you will ever do in your life. You might think that choosing your college, getting married, or buying a house were all major life-changing decisions. And yes, they are big deals, but being a parent is the biggest deal of all. Once you are a parent, you are always a parent. That child is always your child. What that means is different to everyone but nonetheless, it's irreversible. Whether you give birth to that child, whether you have a surrogate, or whether you adopt, you will always be the mother or father of your child.

I am compelled to share my process and clinical experience with you because most patients that I deal with are committed to their diagnosis and have had all their hope obliterated by the mainstream medical community. I am here to say that there is another way. When you are open to getting off the roller coaster, I am happy to take you on a different ride.

New Channel, New Music

"Thank God my doctor told me about you!" This is music to my ears. After 21 years, patients share this sentiment often. Do you know that patients respect a doctor who is current and educated on integrative methods? It's true. I have patients on a daily basis tell me how grateful they are to have been referred to my practice by their medical doctor. This is a dream come true for many patients and certainly for me. Take the best of western medicine and Chinese medicine and offer that to the patients.

Chinese medicine has been treating fertility issues for over 3500 years. Isn't it reasonable to assume that this knowledge could be of value to patients? I sure thought it was! I have educated myself and mainstream medical physicians about Chinese medicine so that more and more patients benefit. It's exciting, it works, and it's accessible.

The Stories

I have patients tell me their stories every day in clinic. They are convinced that they have old eggs, poor quality eggs, and unhealthy uteruses that can't support a pregnancy. They are overwhelmed with the medical jargon and costs (financial, time, and emotional) involved in trying to create a family. Why is this happening to them and what did they do wrong?

How is it possible that so many Hollywood actresses have babies in their late 30s and 40s and I can't get pregnant at 31? Why would I ever think that I would have a problem? It's rarely shared that many famous actresses go through rounds of IVF (in vitro fertilization) cycles that cost tens of thousands of dollars many times over to create their families. Many famous people hire surrogates to carry their pregnancies so their bodies don't go through the weight gain and hormonal cycles that are all a part of pregnancy. This information is not shared and publicized because it's *Hollywood*! It's not real life for you and me. It's smoke and mirrors and the one percent.

You are my typical patient and you are the one that I have been helping for the past 21 years. You get to enjoy the sacred process of being a parent and calling forth life. It does not have to be a nightmare, it doesn't have to hurt, and it doesn't have to ruin your life in the process.

Miracles

In the following chapters I will outline a process that I call a miracle. Why a miracle? A miracle is something that we can't explain. It defies science, logic, and data. There is no repeatable process. We cannot explain it and repeat it at will. A miracle defies all the odds. Miracles are heart-centered. Miracles are soul-driven and deeply felt. Miracles are created in the space between the known and unknown. It's all the stuff that we don't even know we don't know! This is the true meaning of a miracle. I will share in the second chapter my story. My miracle. It's not all hoodoo voodoo either. It's real life. Trust me, I'm a huge skeptic. If I can't touch it, taste it, see it, or smell it, I do not believe it! I am a very results-oriented person and I would never be able to come to work day after day, year after year, without having great results. I don't need to know how every single thing works, I just need to know that it works!

In Chapter Three, I will lay out a plan and help you reconnect with your *instinct*. Your real guide. Instinct tends to get shut down and silenced on the roller-coaster ride when in fact that's exactly where you should be accessing guidance from. You have a deep-seated compass and voice that you get to reconnect with and trust. Your connection with your internal voice or instinct will be your greatest asset in creating your head game.

Chapter Four will be about getting *real*. We will look at lifestyle and how all the small choices are *really* influencing your fertility. We will do a lifestyle assessment and look at all the working pieces. It's going to be fun. It's not good or bad; it's really just getting clear and real.

Chapter Five will be your "A" game plan. You will have an actionable plan to have physiological changes occur. We will talk about sleep and daily habits that are helping and harming. I will offer up solutions and ideas to help you do better and feel healthier.

Chapter Six is about *clarity*. How do we get your body to say "yes" to fertility? How do we really get the body to relax enough so the hormones balance and say yes to ovulation, fertilization, and pregnancy? We'll discuss the science and what we really do know. It's fascinating and brilliant. I love the human body and I can't wait to share the little pearls I've learned over the past 21 years.

Chapter Seven will be a nice *learning* for you. We will learn about whole food nutrition, diet, and some of the successful protocols that we have used for years in our practice.

Chapter Eight will be about *elimination* and *empowerment*. Let's eliminate the fear and myths that tend to keep us stuck during the process. I will break down a lot of the medical jargon and dogma that freaks you out and help you reconnect with the powerful mama you were meant to be. Let's deactivate the "*tick tock tick tock* biological clock time bomb."

Chapter Nine is all about *staying the course*. This is the best training ever for being a parent. It is a rigorous commitment that has no set hours. Some days will be a ten and some days will suck so bad they won't even get on the scale. Obstacles are unavoidable. You got this! I'll share some of the processes and exercises that have helped my patients over the years.

Chapter Ten will offer you the opportunity to get off the roller coaster. You will have a greater understanding of the bigger picture that influences your fertility. You will know that you have options and choices. You will have an opportunity to take this information and run with it and do something different. You will also have an opportunity to work with me one on one.

Only you will know if this speaks to you and your dream of creating a family. If you decide to continue reading and something speaks to you at any point, know that you are exactly in the right place for you at this point in your life.

If there is one thing that I could share with you, it would be this: You are the miracle that your parents called forth and created. If you can connect to that on any level, you have the capacity to create the same miracle.

Chapter One

Miracles

Different Stories, Common Longings

My story begins back in my early teens. I had gynecological issues from the very beginning. For as long as I could remember, I suffered terribly with pain and heavy periods. My parents had me at doctors all the time. The doctors had no idea what was going on. It got to a point where I would be taken to the emergency room, blood drawn, urine sample taken, and then receive the Demerol shot. It was my only relief during the first day or two of my cycle. This happened with regularity. I was miserable at least one week out of the month. As I got older, things got worse. My first semester in college, I flew home two days before classes began to undergo emergency exploratory surgery. I had my left ovary and fallopian tube removed and received a confirmatory diagnosis of stage four endometriosis. I had pretty severe endometrial adhesions in my lower pelvic region and apparently my ovary was necrotic (dead due to poor blood supply) and needed to be removed. Whoa! What was going on with me? Here I was all set to start college life and I was back home with a raging scar right above my privates. *Not my plan.* I made peace with the change of plans and healed up over that semester and got back in the game of life as soon as the next semester rolled around.

The Long Road

I had a lot of relief with my cycles after the surgery. Unfortunately, that relief was short-lived. Approximately six months post-surgery, the pain and discomfort started to creep back in. Eventually I was back to the same level of pain as I had been prior to my surgery. Now that I knew what the diagnosis was, I was able to research and learn about my medical condition. Unfortunately, there was no cure for endometriosis. The medical community treated endo with medications. The treatment strategy was suppression and pain relief. They did not understand what caused it and how to cure it. The only cure would be a hysterectomy. I was barely 18! I learned to manage my pain over the years with different medications. I tried the birth control pill and found that it was not a treatment I could handle. I became an emotional disaster; I was reactive, hyper sensitive, and volatile. I tried pain meds. The pain medication would fog my head and make me feel numb, nauseous and exhausted. I also tried medication to suppress my menstrual cycle. I took Lupron at various points in my 20s to completely shut down my estrogen. Lupron was approved by the FDA for the treatment of prostate cancer. It was being prescribed off-label to suppress estrogen in women who were experiencing estrogen-dominant disease presentations like endometriosis. Lupron was administered by my doctor via monthly injection. It cost me $400.00 a month. I was right out of college, making close to nothing, living in New York, and desperately trying to feel good and not miss work around my period. I fought with my insurance carrier for months about covering my drug costs. After eight months of speaking to supervisors and managers, the health insurance company determined that I had a legitimate case and need for my medication. I was reimbursed for the past eight months of Lupron. This was an unbelievable victory for me – a windfall. I was living paycheck to paycheck and trying to start a life. I was encouraged about the relief the Lupron was giving me and relieved that I wasn't going to go broke affording it. Lupron actually put me in a reversible state of menopause. I stopped getting my period and I of course stopped having pain. At a certain point, I would start to experience severe night sweats and insomnia. The night sweats were happy to show up during the day as well. Hot flashes, no sleep, and the long-term effects of estrogen suppression would have me stop my Lupron for many months to balance out the hormones and cool my system off. This cycle went on for years in my 20s. I also had four laparoscopic procedures over a five-year period to help keep the adhesions and scar tissue controlled. By the time I was 28, I was done. I was on a bad roller-coaster ride and I was ready to get off.

It was years of this cycle that broke me down and brought me to a place of desperation. It felt like my whole life was about my period. If I wasn't getting it, I was getting over it. I would be hung over from the medications and slightly panicked about the imminent onset of my cycle. I had a life to create, enjoy, and live. A career to knock out of the ball park and an incredible partner to meet and have a crazy, exciting, long-term life together. What was really going on with me? How could I continue to do this to my body year after year without paying a price? Common sense dictated that it was not healthy or possible to continue like this.

When All Else Fails ... Surrender

My best friend in the world begged me to try Chinese medicine. He had first-hand experience with acupuncture and Chinese herbs in his fight to survive AIDS. I took his advice and found a great practitioner. I did everything my doctor told me to do. I totally surrendered. I took the herbs, I changed my diet, and tweaked my lifestyle. I had acupuncture on a weekly basis and learned to connect and understand the subtle feedback my body was communicating to me. I acknowledged the headaches, the congestion, the constipation, and the restless sleep. I recognized my impatience and irritability and how it was connected to what I ate or didn't eat. I started to understand how all the dots connected. After three months of consistent treatment, my cycles started to calm down. My pain levels went from a ten to a four or five. My overall energy and mood were enhanced and less volatile. After six months of treatment, I remember walking out of treatment and heading to my car in the large parking lot. I recall thinking how fabulous I felt. I remember feeling the energy I had when I was a nine-year-old. When I was nine, I never wanted the sun to set; I wanted to ride my bike and play outside forever; my energy was boundless. Six months into treatment, I felt the same. I had an epiphany. I thought nothing made more sense to me than this medicine. I needed to study this. I needed to learn more about this medicine so I could share it with people.

Something Old; Something New

Within weeks, I enrolled in Chinese medicine school and started classes at night. School was easy for me. I got it. I was able to comprehend and assimilate the western medicine classes. Chinese medicine was like poetry to me. *Yes. Yes. Yes.* I get it. I knew from a very young age that I wanted to be a doctor and/or a writer. I put both of those callings and dreams on the back burner as I became a responsible practical adult. In my first education, I received a bachelor's degree in advertising and business. It was my first major life decision. I decided that I couldn't afford the luxury of declaring English as a major. Post-grad options were to teach English and live paycheck to paycheck until I wrote the best-selling novel that lived inside me. I wanted my creature comforts, so this career path was incongruent. I took a huge pass on medicine because it failed me miserably and I struggled with chemistry. Now all these years later, the right medicine reveals itself to me and I can't say no.

Back in the 90s, most people were clueless about Chinese medicine. There were very few schools and no job opportunities. I didn't care. I knew it was my path. I started school in New York and ended up transferring to a school in south Florida. I realized that if I were going to have to create a practice one patient at a time, I might as well create relationships and connections in a place that was warm and sunny. I also fell madly in love with golf and that confirmed my decision to move to Florida. I wanted to be able to afford to play and to play all year. I wanted to be a good golfer and this is possible when you live in the sunshine state.

The Path That Heals Also Guides

Upon graduation, I set up my practice, building it literally one patient at a time. It was slow going for the first few years. I wasn't that person who stood in Whole Foods and Barnes and Noble trying to give a talk to shoppers. I decided to create talks for doctors. Just like pharmaceutical reps came in with lunch and presentations about new drugs, I came in with lunch and a 3500-year-old medicine! I educated them on when it might be appropriate to refer a patient to me for acupuncture. I shared research and clinical examples. Some docs thought it was hoodoo voodoo and some thought, oh yeah! Many doctors have thousands of patients they have no idea how to help. They write lots of prescriptions and refer out when the meds don't work. These are my people. I was that patient! As the universe would have it, I attracted a lot of gynecological patients. I became a magnet for PMS, irregular periods, endometriosis, menopausal hot flashes, and fertility patients. I was a research maniac, trying to learn everything I could from both medical lenses. I started to get results with my patients. They in turn shared this info with their medical doctors, creating a circle of belief and trust. I spend every day in practice devoted to creating an environment that offers options and hope for patients.

Obstacles, Longing, and Hopelessness

Back to my miracle and why it matters. I reached a point where I found myself aching to have my child – like you. My path might have been different than yours but the longing was the same. Another childhood dream of mine, besides being a doctor and a writer, was to be a parent. I actually knew from a very young age that I wanted to adopt. I was forever affected by the movie "Oliver." I saw this movie every day for a week when I was visiting my grandparents. Their friend owned the movie theater across the street from their condo. My grandpa walked me across the street at 4 p.m. every afternoon to get a tub of popcorn and Dr. Pepper. I adored Oliver. I couldn't get this movie out of my head. I could never get past the fact that kids were growing up without the love and support of a parent. I promised myself that I would adopt when I got older. The older I got, the stronger and more pressing the desire became.

You might believe that adoption is always an option. In my case, it wasn't. I chose to live my life with another woman in the state of Florida. Back when I was walking the adoption path, it was illegal for gay couples to adopt. *Yes.* People do not believe this fact, but guess what? It's true. This presented lots of obstacles for me. Along with the legal hurdle, I was also facing a relationship hurdle. My partner was not really on board. Having children was not on her radar. She wasn't driven or committed to being a parent. Our lives were great. Why change things? We'd been together for ten amazing years at this point and why rock the boat? It's not as though she was standing in the way of me adopting a child or threatening to leave me if an adoption came to be – she just wasn't investing her energy into the process. As I researched adoption agencies and lawyers and orphanages all over the world, days became months, and months became years. I was getting restless and desperate. I was on the verge of flying to the most AIDS-infested African country to adopt an eight-year-old boy. His medical records were handwritten and emailed to me. They were barely legible. I thought about the long-term ramifications of taking this on. I could bankrupt us. I could have a lifelong medical situation on my hands that would require way more than parenting. I would be taking this child away from his culture, his people, and his friends. I was acting from an irrational emotional state and I was in no position to make life decisions. At least I knew enough to know this!

Taking a Break ... Or So I Thought!

A few months passed and I woke up one day in a start. I told my wife that I needed to go skydiving. She thought I was crazy. I have an unbelievable fear of heights. Why would I want to go skydiving? I can't even snow ski because the fear of hopping off the gondola is paralyzing. I told her that I needed to have a breakthrough. I was frustrated with a new business I was trying to launch outside of my Chinese medicine practice. My thinking was that if I broke through and faced my fear of heights that maybe it would domino into the new business. I would have new insight for the business! Yes, let's do this. Let's not talk about it. Just please set it up and I'll jump. No questions asked. Andrea booked the "breakthrough" adventure for the end of the week. We drove up to Sebastian, Florida on Friday April 20, 2007. We jumped. It was crazy-town amazing. I still remember jumping out of the plane into the fear, fully believing that I was not going to die and that something big was on the other side. We were buzzing from the experience all weekend.

The following Monday morning, we were driving back from our morning walk on the beach, before work when my phone rang. We were sitting at a red light a few blocks from our house. It was about 7:30 a.m. so it was weird to have this friend, who also happens to be a reproductive endocrinologist, call me at this hour. He told me that there was a newborn baby boy that was available for adoption. The adoptive parents backed out at the last minute. He didn't know all the details, but he knew that my patients were open to all options. He also knew that I might be interested. He gave me the number of the attorney handling the case and hung up the phone. I remember it like it was yesterday. I turned to Andrea and repeated the conversation to her. She paused. She is very thoughtful with her words. This morning was no different. She looked me in the eyes and said, "I know that at the end of our lives while we are rocking away on our porch, overlooking the water, that *not* having a child would be the *one* thing in the way of you living your life of no regrets. Call the attorney. I'm in."

This was momentous to say the very least. That morning at 9 a.m., I called the attorney. I passed this attorney's office every day on my drive to my office. *Every single day!* After all the years of "trying" to do this on my own, I had accrued an education about how to handle an adoption contract. I had to legally adopt our son as a single mother. I signed a contract on Monday a.m. I figured that the process would take months. I had heard so many war stories from patients that I believed that I had months, if not years, to get prepared.

The Process

The next morning, Tuesday, I received a call at my office from the attorney telling me that she scheduled a home study for 11 a.m. that morning. I was shocked and excited. I had my office manager reschedule my patients and I headed home. I had no idea what was going to go down in the home study. I had been living with my "wife" for the past ten years and our home was a reflection of that. I mean, we traveled the world and we had pictures all over the place of our amazing moments. I was in a slight panic. We had to de-gay the house! Andrea had to leave for a few hours while our home study was going on. When the doorbell rang at 11 a.m., I opened the door to meet my social worker. I was immediately relieved. She was a "sister" for sure. If you don't know what I mean, then I'll say it straight up. She was gay! She never asked one question about my relationship. She inspected the house to make sure it would be a safe environment to raise a child. She got to know me and my ideas about parenting. It was the fastest two hours of my life. As I walked her out, she looked me in the eye and said, "Get ready, this is going to happen fast." I thought, *yeah right*. I spent the rest of that Tuesday running around Palm Beach county having forms signed and notarized. Every transaction during this day was sprinkled with grace. Windows at government agencies opened when I walked up to them. People were excited and supportive of my urgency to get these papers signed and completed.

Back to Work

The following day was Wednesday. I was scheduled to give a talk in Miami to a Hasidic Jewish organization. It was to a group of rabbis and their wives who counseled couples in their congregation about their fertility issues. Approximately 40 to 50 rabbis flew in for this gathering. I was co-presenting with a close friend who is a reproductive endocrinologist. An east-meets-west mastermind. I had fallen into the fold of this community through patients who found success in my practice. This was another experience laced with grace. My understanding about the talk was that it was going to be an informal Q and A. It ended up that my friend spoke first and he gave a research, pie-chart, statistic-driven PowerPoint presentation. I sat there thinking, *What am I going to say? Chinese medicine? I'm going to speak to a room full of rabbis about acupuncture and herbs?* I was terrified. I just decided at that moment to speak to them like I speak to patients every day. I had nothing to lose. This talk ended up being the most rewarding and connected talk I had given in the ten years I had been practicing. The rabbis were very familiar with Chinese medicine. Judaism and Chinese medicine share a common timeline. I learned that Abraham was an acupuncturist. The thoughtfulness of their questions and their depth of understanding was an unexpected gift. I walked out of that exchange with a full heart.

On my drive home from Miami, I received a call from my attorney. It was 5:45 p.m. and I was in rush hour traffic on I-95. Her exact words, "You can pick your son up. He's yours." Like pick him up tonight? Like the adoption is happening today? We had dinner plans. We had nothing. I mean *nothing* for a newborn. "Really? Tonight?" I regained my composure and told her it would be really stressful to drive to north Florida tonight after I got home. Was it possible to pick him up in the morning? I needed to buy a car seat, a crib, diapers, formula, *everything!*

It Is Happening!

We agreed to arrange pick up from the hospital the following morning. I called Andrea and told her the news. After the initial shock, she began her motherhood experience. She was on her way to Target to get the basics so we could bring our son home. We woke up early and tried to install the car seat. We are two advanced degreed women and we were a huge fail on the car seat install. We headed to the fire department and had Delray's finest help us install our son's first throne. Driving two hours north gave us a little time to dream out loud.

I knew that our son was biracial: half Puerto Rican and half Black American. I knew he was healthy. His birth parents were young and unprepared to raise a child. I decided that I wanted to name him Tiger. I loved Tiger Woods. This of course was before his fall from grace. I still love everything that Tiger did for the game of golf. I loved that he was a hybrid, Asian and Black. I loved his relationship with his parents. I loved that he broke barriers and records in this exclusive, privileged, white man's world. I loved his athleticism, his tenacity, and his creativity. I just loved the idea of Tiger. Andrea was on board. We were on our way to pick up Tiger Lawrence Schiff. Lawrence is Andrea's last name. It was a beautiful name. On the drive up, I called my office and told them the news. I would be out for a few weeks and my schedule needed to be rearranged.

The minute I laid eyes on my son, I fell madly in love. He was finally here. We swaddled him up and took him home. When we arrived at our house, the most heartwarming surprise was waiting for us. Our covered back patio was filled with gifts. Friends and patients had dropped off everything and anything we could ever need for our newborn son. It took my breath away. It is life-changing to really know and feel how much people love and support you. This outpouring of love continued for months. I had a very special patient who had just given birth donate breast milk to Tiger for the first eight months of his life. I had a patient come to my house and set up a Bellini crib that her son had grown out of. There were many moments that I'll never forget.

The Elements Are All Mine; The Longings of the Heart Are the Same

The grace that blessed our lives during this time was pure and purposeful. It was way bigger than we could imagine. This is when I knew for sure that our son chose us and that he was a miracle. I couldn't explain it. I always believed it would happen and I have seen it happen in many ways for many patients. Sometimes, oftentimes our paths are not what we think they are. It doesn't mean our dreams are not coming to fruition.

I want to point out something else. I had been working my adoption process for years. Notice the time frame of how Tiger came to me.

I jumped out of a plane on Friday, April 20. Intent to have a breakthrough. Tiger was born Saturday, April 21, 2007. I received a phone call on Monday, April 23, 2007. I picked him up from the hospital Thursday, April 26, 2007. After years and years of desire and longing, I was blessed with one week of grace. It was like I got the thumbs up from the universe that it was my time.

Babies Come Many Ways

So why is my story important? Why would it matter to you? You're not interested in adoption. Your story is different. You don't have the hurdles I had. Yes. All true perhaps. But we have the same dream. We share the same base guttural longing to be a mom. It's a part of our fabric and birthright that we as women get to be a mom. Some of us must birth our children. Some of us can't fathom childbirth but know we were meant to be a mom. I get the longing, I get the physiological challenges. I empathize with the emotional highs and lows. Every fertility patient in the end wants the same thing. We are all mothers waiting in the wings for our child.

Chapter Two

I Can't Do This Anymore

"I *need* to do something different." I get what this feels like. It's your tipping point. I felt this way after years of hormones, pain killers, and laparoscopic surgeries. It was so clear. I was done and now you are done. You are ready to get off the roller coaster. I realized that what I was doing for so many years was futile. I was buying time. I was wasting time. I was *not* addressing the underlying cause of my imbalance and the path I was on never would. There had to be a better way. After years and years of treatment, education, and clinical experience, I am happy to share all the pearls that I have discovered. I have used my protocols with great success, not only for myself, but for thousands of patients over the past 20 years.

Options, Alternatives, and Opportunities

For some reason, no one has figured out why your body is saying "no" to pregnancy. If they have, they haven't offered up a solution that has worked. If you have miscarried, your body is saying "no" to staying pregnant. My plan is all about getting your body to say "*Yes.*" Your body has an innate intelligence that keeps it humming along under most conditions. Heart is beating, lungs are inhaling and exhaling, hormones are being secreted from organs and glands, and most of us tend to think everything is wonderful until it's not. We tend to think that we are healthy until our bodies don't do what we want or need them to do. One thing that is clear is that pregnancy is a stressor on the body – no matter how old you are and no matter how healthy you think you are. You are asking your body to not only support and regulate all life function for yourself but you are also asking it to support the development of an embryo into a fetus into a full-on, living, breathing human being. All the while keeping you healthy and functional in your everyday busy and demanding life. I believe that the body's priority is survival. Sometimes we just don't get how our lifestyles, stress levels, lack of deep REM sleep, diet, and work interfere with the optimal health of our bodies. Our internal command center chooses *you* over you being at risk. This is a big reason our bodies say *no*.

Five Steps to Increase Your Chances of Your Body Saying "Yes"

In the following chapters, I will lay out a process that I have used for years with great success. The most common side effects are feeling healthier, looking rested and younger, and an overall improvement in your life attitude. Not the usual fine-print, scary side effects that you are used to hearing on drug commercials or reading on prescription drug package inserts. This process is doable and accessible to anyone who is really ready to commit and do something different. You may have dabbled in some of my steps to some degree at some point thus far. This is not my plan. My plan is all in. Let's do this and let's do it now.

Step One: Head Game

Getting your head in the right place is critical. I'm pretty sure this is the most important step. If we can't change our thoughts and reactions to the situations that have gotten us here, then we are more than likely going to struggle and suffer more than we have to. If you're reading this book, you are ready. You are willing to try anything at this point. I'm not suggesting that you need deep psychotherapy or anything like that. I'm just saying that I have heard so many similar thought patterns that drive infertility that I can't ignore the impact that your mind is having on your process. I can help.

Step Two: Lifestyle Assessment

We're going to look at everything! Diet, medications, sleep habits, elimination, drugs, alcohol, exercise, relationships, play time, family, etc.... You name it, we will explore it. If it was just about the sperm and the egg, you would probably be pregnant already. It's eye-opening and life-changing to really widen the lens of your life and see how you are taking care of your body. Many women don't even need a lot of help when they see the patterns that have them feeling not so fabulous. We will also explore your health history and family history. This is all about you and how to get your body to say yes.

Step Three: Action

Step Three is all about an actionable plan. We will explore diet ideas and realistic choices to enhance your fertility. You will also walk away from this step having a greater understanding of the liver from a western and Chinese medicine perspective. I have seen a lot of great success with hormone imbalance and fertility enhancement once the liver is functioning optimally. We'll explore exercise options and how and why certain practices are draining and depleting as opposed to those that are supplementing and restorative. You will have action steps that you can implement at the end of this chapter.

Step Four: Circadian Rhythm

Understanding your circadian rhythm is life changing. I will break down the basics when it comes to right timing. After all, isn't timing everything in life? It's actually everything in creating life too! Most of us are disconnected to the inherent cycles that rule our life cycle. This information will rock your world. You'll begin to connect the dots about your recurrent November cough, your full moon insomnia, and your annual summer eczema outbreak. Awareness and connection to your strengths and weaknesses affords you a fighting chance to improve your overall health and of course, your fertility.

Step Five: Lab Values and All the Medical Jargon

Understanding the lab values can change your head game. If you can change your head game, you will change your entire experience. So many of us walk around thinking we are our lab values and our diagnosis. This doesn't serve us and, in many situations, it hurts us. Deeply. This step will break it all down and allow you to separate the fact from the fiction. There is a lot of medical jargon, fancy names, and acronyms that stand for complicated procedures. We get to just dumb it down and digest it so it doesn't paralyze or scare us.

I know you've been through your own personal nightmare and you are ready to open another door and walk through it. No matter where you are in your fertility path, I can assure you this: You will get through this. I promise. More than likely, this was never your plan. You probably went to great efforts to *not* get pregnant when you were younger. No one plans to be here. Now that you are, let's do this in the healthiest way possible. Whether you are looking to improve your chances of conceiving naturally, or with IVF or surrogacy, this plan will support your process. This plan might even help you open the gates of adoption. Having a child and being a parent is the most important thing you might ever do in this life. I am here to get you there in the healthiest way I know how.

I will leave you with this anecdote from years of working with patients just like you. The more conditional you are about how your child has to come to you, the more contractive you become. Think about that and what that might mean for you. When a patient has a life plan and this baby thing is not following the plan – this is a contractive space. Like my plan was to go to college, grad school, and then land a job at a big brokerage house, date, meet a great guy, and then, in like two years, get pregnant with my first and then have another two years later. Very contractive when it doesn't happen like that. The more attached you are to plans like this, the greater likelihood you are in a state of contraction.

Remember all the guys you dated before you met your husband? All the bad dates and awkward phone calls and texts? Remember thinking, "Oh my God, when will I ever meet a guy that I can get serious about?" And then he kind of shows up when you least expect it. It all worked out somehow. Even when you never thought it would. This is a similar life situation. It's bittersweet and definitely uncomfortable, but I am encouraging you to be brave, take a deep breath, and trust that you will find your way through to the other side.

Real Patient Story

Marcella came to see me about nine years ago. She was, like you, *done*. Although her story details are all her own, she was, like you, at her rope's end. Marcella was a foreign language professor at a local university. She taught multiple classes all week and was doing research and writing papers for her upcoming tenure approval. In between her rigorous work demands, she ran to doctors and appointments trying to uncover the reasons she and her husband were not getting pregnant. It all started out slowly. First a few rounds of Clomid with timed intercourse, followed by several rounds of Clomid and IUIs (inter-uterine inseminations.) She became pregnant two times during her Clomid period, but unfortunately miscarried both times. They were early miscarriages so the doctors weren't too concerned. Miscarriage is very common. After a few more months of failed procedures, Marcella decided to take a summer break and look for a new doctor in the fall.

She travelled to Europe with her students to chaperone a six-week language immersion. She returned reinvigorated and ready to start up again. She began treating with another IVF clinic and they fast tracked her right into an IVF cycle. The IVF cycle was very intrusive in her tight schedule. She had to be monitored every other morning at the clinic. The clinic was 25 minutes from her office. The wait time in the clinic was unpredictable. It was filled with working "want-to-be mothers" all freaking out about being late and getting bad news after their ultrasound. It didn't even have to be bad news. It could be no news and a "look" from the sonographer that the woman perceived as bad. The elevated hormone levels in the IVF waiting room were intense and short-fused. The sensitivity scale was a 19 on the one to ten scale. Marcella went on to go through four consecutive IVF cycles. She got pregnant twice and miscarried again both times. By the time she came to treat with me, she was spent. Three years of doctors, clinics, hormones, procedures, poking, prodding, and four miscarriages … her gas tank was empty. The moment we sat in consultation, I felt her pain and depletion. She wanted my help in getting her health back. She said that the past three years knocked the life out of her. She was in no position to consider having a baby until she felt like a person again.

Surrender

Health became her priority. She taught for the past 20 years and there was no way she wasn't going to get her tenure because of health complications. More than that, she wanted to enjoy the comfort of having her tenure while doing what she loved. Marcella was, as you might imagine, an extremely compliant patient. I laid out a realistic plan to detox her, and then nourish her up. She started to come back to life after about three months. The light in her eyes started to slowly shine and connect. Her skin cleared up and her bloating and fatigue began to fade. After six months of care, Marcella was getting ready to head to Europe with her students. It was summer again and classes were done and she was feeling well enough and even excited to travel.

Two months passed before I saw Marcella on my schedule again. I walked up to my reception area getting ready to take the next patient and I saw that it was Marcella. She was back. She was different. Her energy was lit up. I walked her back to a treatment room and the minute I closed the door she told me the news. "I'm pregnant. Almost four and a half months! I realized when I was in Europe but I didn't want to get excited because of all the prior losses. I just decided to enjoy my summer and then when I got home, I was scared to go to the doctor. I felt great and I didn't want to hear any bad news. Finally, my husband convinced me to go to my ob-gyn. He confirmed that I was pregnant and that the baby was about four and a half months old. I heard the heartbeat and I saw him! It's a boy."

Marcella went on to have a wonderful pregnancy. She gave birth to a beautiful healthy boy. She recovered well and was able to enjoy her maternity leave and bond with her son. She continued under my care throughout the year. Marcella returned to work and continued to maintain her healthy habits. She became pregnant again, *naturally*, 18 months after her first son was born. She was a little bit busier this pregnancy with a toddler added to her tenure-approved teaching life, but she enjoyed another healthy pregnancy and gave birth to another gorgeous chunky boy.

I share this story because it really happened. It may seem extreme or it may very much be like your story. It doesn't have to be this extreme. Your "surrender point" might come sooner. It might come later. The bottom line is that the healthier you are, the greater chance you will have at having your body say yes. I never mentioned the small fortune that this patient spent on medications and high-tech procedures. My concern is always a patient's health. But I know as well as you that financial pressure wreaks havoc on your stress and anxiety meter. This in turn has a direct effect on your physical health.

I am going to share a patient story in each chapter, just to remind you that you are not on this ride alone. Infertility is widespread and non-discriminating. So, if you're ready to dive into the five steps that will give your body the best chance of saying yes, let's go!

Chapter Three

Instinct and Intuition and Your Inner Voice

Wow, how long has it been since you've had a date with your intuition? Do you remember? I know for years I was on complete disconnect with my "gut feeling" and inner voice. I, like you, believed that the doctors knew best. Of course. They go to school forever, they specialize and they understand. Right? Isn't that what most people think? Now you don't even have to leave your home. You can access Dr. Google anytime you want. Five in the morning, midnight, and all-day Sunday. Dr. Google and infertility chat groups will provide all the medical advice you could ever dream of. You could also lose your mind and all your free time spiraling down the rabbit hole of the internet.

What if you didn't need to ask anyone or go anywhere? What if you could just understand what your next step is going to be by being still? I know you think everyone else knows better and that someone is going to have the "right" answer to make everything all better, but the reality is that you have the answers. I know you are struggling. I know you are frustrated, sad, overwhelmed, depressed, and angry. I know. I feel it from you. Yes, I am saying that you might need some help and support but not at the expense of shushing up your inner voice.

In most cases, infertility will afford you time to be alone. Sometimes you might feel like it's too much time. Like you are pulling back from social situations and other people's happy life events. It's difficult to be social and excited for coworkers and friends who are pregnant and celebrating births, baby showers, baby naming parties, brises, and christenings. It's like salt on your wounded heart. It's OK.

Choices

So, in these times when you are alone, it's easy to rehash and relive everything you've done up until this point. The choices that you made that have gotten you here. The choice to wait until you met the right man. The choice you made to be on birth control the majority of your ovulating life. The choice you made to terminate a pregnancy when you were 20 and in college on your pre-law school track. The choice you made to take Depo injections so you wouldn't have to even deal with having a period because it was too annoying to deal with. The choice you made to not look into the fact that you have never had a regular menstrual cycle your entire life even though you kind of knew this wasn't exactly normal. All the choices you made that you spin into stories about making this fertility nightmare your fault and some kind of payment or punishment. Yeah, this is definitely *not* the best use of your head space.

You may also be creating a whole production about this period of your life being someone else's fault. That's just as big as "your-fault" stories. The most common story I hear is the bad doctor story. Another one is it's the media's fault. Who would have thought I would have a problem at 35 when Celine Dion is having twins at 42? My grandmother had my mother when she was 40. My cousin in Wyoming had kids into her mid-forties. Or, my husband never wanted kids when we were younger and now that he's ready, we can't.

There are endless reasons that you can come up with that will support your stories about why there is a reason to blame yourself or someone else – for your fertility or for anything in life. It's especially relevant to those things you really want and think you deserve. I am inviting you to release the game of blame and fault-finding and invest in the game of intuition and instinct.

Shhhhhhhhhhhhhhhhh ... Listen

It's time to reconnect with what you really need to hear. You are at that point where you get to rekindle your relationship with your inner knowing and your inner guide. Your gut feelings. You know that feeling when you walked out of the "specialist's" office after he laid out a bunch of scary statistics about how old your eggs were at 37 and the chances of having a normal baby at your age were about 2 percent on your own but with a $30,000 donor egg IVF cycle you would have your best chance of having a baby? You know that feeling you had when he escorted you to the finance manager and scheduler on the way out? You know that state of shock (that is actually your internal *pause* button) you were in with an undercurrent of "this doesn't feel right" trying to reach your vocal cords? This is your intuition. Your inner knowing. You know when you are injecting yourself with hormones, putting patches on your body, and timing every bodily discharge and sex act and nothing feels good or right for you? This is your intuition. You know that feeling when you decide to go to a conveniently located chiropractor who also does acupuncture and you feel like they have no clue about infertility but you rationalize that at least you're doing acupuncture and insurance pays for it? Yeah, that's your intuition. Would you go to an orthopedist to have your tooth pulled? Trust your instinct.

I have seen too many patients surrender their common sense and intuition to bad medical practice. I am talking about really smart, successful, powerful women! The tops in their fields. Big breadwinners, game changers, and leaders, all giving up their inner knowing. This process is rooted in that deepest yin aspect of being a woman. Yin is a Chinese medicine term: yin and yang. Yin refers to the deep core of creation. The dark space within. The root of all intention and life. Yang is the manifestation of yin. It is the action, motion, and expression of the yin. They are thunder and lightning. Symbiotic and interconnected. In lay terms, if you completely disconnect from your inner voice and yin core, it's difficult to manage the journey. It will increase your odds of disconnection and unhappiness.

Creating a healthy head game will increase your odds of having a baby and creating a family. The first step in this process is to get to know your inner voice. If you are at the point that you are reading this book, you must have had a conversation or two with her already. That is perfect. First of all, you need to know that she is your best friend. She's looking out for you. She has competition all the time from the other voices that talk louder. You know those voices … fear, guilt, shame, and doubt. They all live in the "not-good-enough" file in your hard drive! Not sure how we all seem to have that file. It's kind of like the apps that you can't delete from your laptop and phone without crashing the system. Is there really something you can do to nourish and restore that inner voice? Yes, there is.

Nourishing and fertilizing your instinct and inner knowing is a critical starting point. First off, it's really important to talk to her. You can do this through writing. You can do this by having a conversation out loud or in your own head. If you are techy, you could actually video yourself talking to her. You can talk to a picture of yourself. This picture represents your highest, most loving self: the most yin aspect of yourself. The little girl dreamer who knows that anything is possible. Ask yourself the hard questions. The ones that you can't begin to say out loud. This will lay the ground work for everything going forward, so don't hold back. No one needs to ever read this or see what you've said or written. I'm talking about questions like, "Why do I really want to have a baby? Will I be a good mother? Can I really handle birthing a baby? Will my husband still be attracted to me after I'm pregnant and give birth? Can we really afford a baby? Are we emotionally ready for this? Can our relationship bear the pressure of a child? How will I know if my baby will be healthy? What if I don't love my baby? What if my baby is ugly? Is my husband really the person I want to raise my child?" I know these questions sound crazy to some of you and to others they might be exactly what you are thinking. Every one of us has our own questions that we are unwilling to ask and answer. I promise you, if you take the time to be quiet and thoughtful and honest with yourself, your questions will bubble up. When they do, know that you have an opportunity to break through. You will be entering into that relationship with your inner knowing, instinct, and intuition. This is your home base and you can never go wrong operating from here.

Staying connected to your inner voice takes practice, especially when she's been ignored for long periods of time. Now that you have established a connection, only you will know how strong and accessible the connection is. I personally like to be connected all the time. I always trust my inner voice and instinct and I like to have 24/7 access. Some of the greatest interruptions in this relationship are static and noise. Background noise like traffic, voices, televisions, phones, computers, trains, planes, and even food! Always being in the doing. Strenuous exercise – I call it yang exercise. The kind of exercise that has you numb out and flood the system with endorphins at first and then exhaust you. It's like a distraction from yourself. I love yang exercise, but I also alternate with yin yoga, tai chi, and meditation. Meditation is a tough practice for many people. I get it. It can appear to be unproductive, boring, and useless. Until you do it with regularity and reap the benefits, it's a tough enrollment. Meditation is free and you don't need any equipment or special clothes. You can do it anywhere. You don't need a degree or need to know the right people. You don't need to be a certain age and you don't need a partner. It's like the Visa commercial. It's priceless. It's a space to connect to your inner voice and the universe all in one. I recommend this as a non-negotiable in creating your head game.

Another valuable addition to nourishing your head game and inner self-talk would be to surround yourself with podcasts, meditations, and mantras that support you. The internet has made it possible to access great programs that are very budget-friendly or free. You can subscribe to

Headspace, download Circle and Bloom, and/or Organic Conceptions. I have many patients who listen to these recordings or meditations during their treatments. You can carve out 20 to 30 minutes a day to bathe your intuitive inner self with some fertilizing juju. Whether you do a guided meditation, Transcendental meditation, or a group meditation, I can assure you that this regular practice will benefit your overall health, fertility, and outlook on life.

In the process of creating a solid head game, sometimes it's super comforting and helpful to have a fertility buddy. I know this sounds hokey, but fertility buddy connections have been made for years in the reception area of my office. These relationships can be invaluable. I know women who have created lifelong connections during this process. As unique and wonderfully special as you might be, I need to let you know that there are others going through the same thing. Be open to making a connection. When you are on this path, it can be lonely and isolating and to have the understanding and friendship of another woman on the same road can be lifesaving. I recommend this with an ounce of caution. You are looking to connect with someone who is also looking to up her head game. Meeting people who are willing to bring you down and share their rotten attitude and wallow in blame and fault stories is *not* a good match. You're moving in a different direction.

Instinct and intuition are also not bound by limitations. I want you to think about this. When I was faced with my relentless monthly painful periods and the limitations of western medicine, I felt boxed in. Like I could suffer or be drugged. Or if I really wanted to go for broke, I could have a hysterectomy. I rationally believed that these were my three options and that was *it*. It took me years to reach the point where I was completely desperate and ready to surrender. My inner knowing was raging to be heard. There had to be another way. I knew what I was doing was not healthy. I rarely felt good and I couldn't accept this. I had so much to do in this world and not being healthy just wasn't an option. You could have *never* told my 25-year-old self that I would be writing this book after practicing Chinese medicine for over 20 years. Never! I would never have been able to wrap my head around that thought. Everything that you have chosen and done up until this point is what you obviously should have been doing. You are here now. And now you get to reconnect and listen. Trust. It's in those moments that you see the lightning, and instead of covering your ears, you embrace the thunder. Options appear just when you thought you were out of them. The deal is this though … they were always there. You just couldn't see them.

Let's recap. Connecting with your inner knowing, instinct, and intuition is a critical first step in creating your head game. Make a habit of connecting with your instinct until it becomes a constant state. Your fastest route to this connection in my experience is being still and meditating. Ask yourself your hard questions. Whatever they are. Nothing is off limits. After you ask these questions, allow yourself to answer them honestly. No editing. Get it all out. You more than likely will feel some relief. You also might feel greater clarity about where you are.

Consider downloading some guided meditations. They don't even need to be about fertility. Anything that settles down your monkey brain and helps you connect to your inner self is perfect. What resonates with you today might change in six weeks. Go with it. There is no right way to do this. Consider swapping a spin class for yin yoga or tai chi once or twice a week.

Lastly, if this resonates for you, consider opening yourself up to a fertility buddy. If you set that intention and ask for support from people in your life, you might be surprised how many women are looking to connect with you. Many women are having fertility issues. Everyone knows someone who is doing IVF, had a miscarriage, has PCOS, and is having difficulty creating a family. If you're looking for a buddy, I can assure you she's looking for you.

Chapter Four

Lifestyle Assessment

Yes, we need to get into this. There's just no way to not talk about this. I am going to break things down so it makes sense. In the process you might have some *aha* moments. Some things may hit home and others won't. I can tell you that all the small choices add up. This is great news for you because small changes over time will deliver big results.

Before I talk about lifestyle assessment, I want to explain a scary sounding term. Please try to stick with this so you understand the power you have to make your body healthier and, in turn, more fertile. The term I want to discuss is follicular genesis. No, this is not a section of the bible! This is a brilliant female reproductive function.

Imagine this: When you are about four to five months in utero (developing in your mommy's belly), you develop all the follicles you will ever have. What's a follicle? A follicle houses the egg that, when fertilized, creates the miracle of life. By the time you are born, it is guesstimated that you have about one to two million follicles. By the time you begin menstruating, you are down to about 300,000 follicles.

What does all this mean? If you really think about it, your mother's health has had some influence on the health of your follicles in utero. If you really want to trip out, you will realize that your grandmother's health had an impact on your health, because your mother's follicles were bathed in the placenta your grandmother created. It's really trippy to think about these things!

Okay, so how does it all work and how can you improve it? When I say "it," I am referring to your egg quality reserve. Every month, your ovaries recruit the best of the best from your reserves to potentially be ovulated. You might have had a trans-vaginal ultrasound at some point and the nurse said, "Oh, look you have four on the left and seven on the right." You will ovulate one of those follicles upon hormonal trigger. The most dominant follicle will break out from the ovary and find its way into your fallopian tube. As it travels down toward the uterus there is a chance for that egg to become fertilized and implant into the endometrial lining. The other follicles that did not ovulate go through a process of atresia and die. Every month, an ovulating woman recruits the best of the best from her follicular reserve from her ovaries. These follicles are now in the possible pool of ovulation. This process of recruitment happens over a period of three to four months. The good news is that you can really impact the health of your reserve over a three- to four-month period.

Sometimes I think of the process like baseball. There are major league players, minor league players, and many training camps and lower league players that work hard to get recruited up to the majors. All of these lower league players are training hard and improving their potential in the hopes of being chosen for the chance to play major league ball. These up and comers don't only play baseball. They train in the gym, they work on their head game, they do drills, eat high quality diets, and rehab when injured. Their body is their temple. In order to play in the majors, they have a game plan. This is a parallel universe to your egg quality. You can nourish and improve the environment and nutrient infusion to your eggs in many small ways over time.

My hope for you is to no longer be overwhelmed or feel powerless when you hear medical terminology like follicular genesis. All it means is egg recruitment. More than 70 percent of the patients who come to work with me are convinced that their eggs are old and the ones that are left are lousy. Let's throw that thought out and see what we can do to create a new thought.

Treating the Masses

You know that Western medicine has set up protocols and treatment parameters to be able to treat the masses. No matter what your labs reveal, if you have been trying to conceive for over a year, and you are 35 or older, a reproductive endocrinologist will tell you that you have egg quality concerns. Yes, it's true that chronological age is a variable, but with that being said, most women can and will conceive. We see it clinically year after year.

A lifestyle assessment can provide clarity and help you make better choices. I talked earlier about how your body has an innate intelligence. Your body will always prioritize how it uses its resources. When I talk about resources I am referring to blood. I am referring to qi (pronounced chi). For sake of ease, let's just translate qi into energy. The lack of or abundance of energy you feel on a daily basis is the qi I'm referring to. This distribution of blood and qi is used internally for all bodily functions. Your body decides to drive blood flow and energy to your gut to digest, your brain to think and to influence hormones. Your body uses qi to pump blood through your circulatory system and to your liver to filtrate out the toxins, preservatives, and all the additives in our water, food, and atmosphere. Qi and blood are used to support the kidneys, small intestine, bladder, and bowels. And lastly, our body uses qi and blood to nourish our reproductive organs to procreate. As discussed earlier, your body's priority is survival, not reproduction. *So* how do we get your body to say yes? How do we move out of survival into an optimal fertile state?

Lifestyle choices are always something we have the option to change and improve. Diet is a big concern. Stress is also big concern. I am talking about stressful work situations, stressful friendships, and stressful family dynamics. Long commutes that have you rigid and contracted and on high alert two hours a day, five days a week are a contributing factor. Lack of sleep or light sleep can be a big variable in your optimal hormonal function. Alcohol, cigarettes, and recreational drug use will influence egg and sperm quality. I won't waste your time with research here because it's all available on the internet. Let's assume this is all common knowledge. It is not beneficial or helpful pretending that these choices don't matter. I promise you they do.

All the Small Choices Add Up

When I work with you as a patient, one of the first things I do is have you fill out a journal. We supply the journal and we like you to return it after a two-week period. This journal is a record of food and fluid intake, plus sleep habits and quality of sleep, bowel movements, mood, and energy. The fact is, most patients want acupuncture and an herbal prescription and to continue what they have been doing all along. This is not a successful strategy. Acupuncture treatments are 30 minutes. Even if a patient comes in twice a week, that's a total of one hour of treatment. There are 168 hours in a week. I can assure you that all the small choices you are making in the other 167 hours are critical to how your body is using its resources, meaning where your body decides to send your qi and blood.

During this period of becoming conscious of how you are feeding, resting, and emotionally nourishing your body, there is a general awareness that starts to reveal itself. When you start coming off of autopilot and hold yourself accountable to just writing things down, it's impossible to not have a wakeup call. I remember doing this for myself just to understand what small choices I was making on a daily basis.

Just a Spoonful of Sugar

I realized that I was having two cups of coffee a day. I put two teaspoons of sugar in each cup. I decided that four teaspoons of sugar, seven days a week, 52 weeks a year, was way too much sugar. This was only the sugar in my coffee! I did not want to think about the other ways I routinely consumed sugar. I decided to reduce my conscious sugar consumption over a month. By the end of four weeks, I was drinking one cup of coffee with one teaspoon of sugar. I went from consuming 1460 teaspoons of sugar to 365 teaspoons of sugar over a year. That's a whole lot of sugar! I have to say, I felt better. I actually never felt bad. When I eliminated that extra cup and three teaspoons of sugar on a daily basis, I really felt terrific. We all know the impact sugar has on inflammation, diabetes, and cancer, so how can you not think that small changes over long periods of time could not help improve your fertility? I know it can.

I will share my thoughts and suggestions in the next few chapters. I know there is a lot of conflicting information on what to eat and what not to eat. I will make it simple and realistic. Changing your diet is one of the most difficult lifestyle habits people struggle with. It doesn't have to be difficult. I will tell you that if you are fast-fooding your way through the week, that will have to change. Think of it like this: One day you would like to retire. I am sure you are not thinking that at 65 you will have all of a sudden receive a check that will support you for the rest of your life. If you are like most of us, you have a plan in place. You are saving or investing a little bit at a time to help support yourself when that time comes. Your health deserves *at least* this amount of this thought and consideration. The reality is that saving for retirement is all for naught if you don't have your health. The same thinking applies to your fertility. The healthier you are going into a pregnancy, the greater likelihood your body will say yes to fertility.

Real Patient Story

Kelly was dying to have a baby. She and her husband had been trying for several years and now that she was 34, she was feeling the crunch of the ticking biological clock. Her regular gynecologist wanted her to go to a specialist but she wasn't on board for all that high-tech doctoring. Kelly was a school administrator with a lot of responsibility. She drove 45 minutes each way to her office. It was the price she was willing to pay to live in a less congested area that had larger parcels of land. Her big dream was to have a house full of kids and a big yard for them to play in.

Kelly had an obvious case of poor nutrition and exhaustion. She was a light and interrupted sleeper. She never felt well-rested when she woke up. Even on the weekend when she slept in, she still felt exhausted. Her diet was a combination of drive-through McDonalds, Wendy's, or Dunkin Donuts. Lunch was usually the school cafeteria or vending machines. She loved her Coke and flavored coffee creamers. The weekend evenings were spent with friends at restaurants and comedy clubs. After grinding all week, it was common to drink three or four glasses of wine or beer. Her husband was a bourbon guy.

On further examination, Kelly revealed that her cycles were really heavy, clotty, and painful. She had to take pain medication the day before and after her cycle began. Sometimes she missed work. She also suffered from painful varicose veins in her legs and hemorrhoids. She always knew when her cycle was coming because she would get her monthly headache. It was her "period-is-coming" headache. Three Advils every four hours usually did the trick. This is how Kelly's periods had been for many years now, so she thought all these symptoms were normal. I told her it may be common but it was not optimal or a reflection of health.

Once Kelly reviewed her lifestyle assessment with me, she was very aware of how she could do better. She decided that she would do whatever I suggested because it made perfect sense that her body was saying no for obvious reasons. We detoxed her with herbs and dietary changes and started her on a program to move and facilitate healthy blood flow through her circulatory system. She made time for food shopping and food prep, acupuncture, meditation, and mild but moving exercise. Her periods began to change over a three-month period. Her monthly headaches were gone and her pain level decreased to the point where she no longer took Advil or missed work. She lost 18 pounds over a four-month period, *just by eliminating processed food*. Kelly became pregnant, naturally, after seven months of making small changes and sticking to them.

I wish I had before and after pictures of this woman. Since I tend to work with fertility, most of the time I forget how much a healthy lifestyle can influence hair, skin, and overall vitality. She was a different woman. Kelly gave birth to healthy boy after a normal pregnancy. The varicose veins and hemorrhoids started to come to life again toward the end of her pregnancy but she addressed them with herbs and recovered within weeks. Kelly had two more boys over the next three years. All naturally. She finally stopped trying for a girl when she realized her life was stretched to capacity. She comes in from time to time for a tune up and a reassessment of her health. She has learned to make better choices for herself post-partum and for her children.

I'm not saying that by eliminating fast food you will automatically become pregnant. That would be ludicrous. I am saying that an overall lifestyle assessment can reveal areas that can be improved and in turn influence your chance of your body saying yes to becoming pregnant.

Chapter Five

Diet, Whole Food Nutrition, and Supplements

Ugh … the "D" word. Diet. It has so much baggage. It implies restriction and denying yourself the good stuff. Most of my patients are confused about what to eat. There is so much conflicting information. I get it. I am a baby boomer and I was raised during the Sweet'n Low era heyday. We have seen higher rates of obesity and diabetes since artificial sweeteners and low-fat foods monopolized mainstream media. I like to make this part of my program as simple and accessible as possible. None of us needs to be stressed out about what we are eating.

After you complete the two-week journal of your lifestyle habits, eating habits become obvious. Just like I cut down on sugar in my coffee over a four-week period, I was able to see the impact those small choices produced over an extended period of time. Moderation is always going to be a fallback strategy for me. There is nothing moderate about our consumption habits. Supersize, double patties, and grandes are a part of our daily menu choices. I want to encourage you to think about moderation. Moderation and balance are going to serve you in the long run.

Before we get into what to eat, I want to explain another process I suggest patients do when they work with me. Most of my patients are highly motivated and ready to do whatever it takes to get their body to say yes. I am usually not the first stop along their journey. I usually see patients after failed cycles or after trying different products and supplements they found on the internet or in the fertility section in a health food store. People take a lot of lousy products that are loaded with fillers. It dawned on me years ago that my patients needed a good purification before we started nourishing them with great food choices and nutrition.

Oh My Liver!

This is how and why we encourage patients to do a 21-day liver purification as a first step. Do you know what the liver does in your body? The liver has hundreds of functions but there are four major functions that I like to bring to light.

Number one: The liver is a major filtration organ. The liver initiates filtration of everything you put into your body. Every medication, synthetic hormone, preservative, pesticide, alcohol, and chemical element gets filtrated through the liver.

Number two: The liver synthesizes hormones. This means that the liver plays a role in having our hormones function efficiently. If you are experiencing any hormone imbalance, clearing and fortifying your liver function is critical. Understanding this is pivotal. Because the liver synthesizes hormones, it's going to have an impact on your thyroid, your pancreas, and your ovaries. All three of these organs secrete hormones that are essential to your body saying "absolutely yes" to fertility. I will guestimate that at least 70 percent of the patients I see are on some form of thyroid support. Most patients have a history of long term birth control use. I also treat many patients that have a history of Adderall and Ritalin-type meds as well as anti-depressants. Couple all of this with alcohol, processed food, and everyday stressors, and you can understand how much work your liver has been up to.

So why are the liver values on your labs normal? Just because your lab values are in range does not mean that you are healthy or optimal. Do you know that you have to be down to 14 percent function of your kidneys in order to be diagnosed with kidney failure? I am all about being proactive and about preservation. Who wants to wait until the wheels fall off?

Number three: The liver converts 80 percent of T4 to T3. OK, what the heck does this mean? T4 and T3 are your primary thyroid hormones. Most of you are familiar with TSH. TSH (thyroid stimulation hormone) stimulates the secretion of T4 and T3 from the thyroid gland. T4 means four molecules of iodine. T3 means three molecules of iodine. Cells use T3. T4 is in the wings waiting for the need to be converted to T3. When the demand is there the liver will convert T4 to T3, *if the liver is functioning efficiently.* What is the big deal with the thyroid anyway? Every organ and gland in the body needs a little bit of thyroid hormone to turn on. If the thyroid is not functioning well, it can make everything drag and stagnate. There is also a relationship between recurrent pregnancy loss and thyroid dysfunction. Cleaning up the liver can and will influence your thyroid efficiency.

Number four: The liver produces cholesterol. Cholesterol is the building block for hormones. We need and want healthy hormone production. Cholesterol is not a dirty word. Like all other levels in our labs, it is something to consider watching. I never look at levels and make a final assumption about a patient. I look for patterns. I look for inter relationships of levels and how they are expressing a burden on a system. I look for inflammatory markers in addition to cholesterol levels because cholesterol alone is not significant to me. If I see hypothyroidism, insulin resistance, and high FSH levels, you better believe a liver purification is step one.

Our liver purification protocol is not difficult. I work with the oldest whole foods nutrition company in the United States and they package a simple program with a ton of support. You can access recipes and food planning on their site. The basic premise is *clean* eating while you are detoxing and fortifying your system. A simple principle to keep in mind is twice as many veggies as fruit. We tweak the program for the individual patient but the program can work for anyone. After understanding the impact the liver has on the body, I started doing the liver purification annually. I usually do it from November 1 – the day after Halloween – through the three weeks before Thanksgiving; twenty-one days is perfect. This process gets me into a conscious state about how I am feeding myself and how I am feeling. It is a great strategy to manage all the temptation over the holidays.

After the purification, you will be ready to start taking some high quality nutritional support and actually benefit from them. Now that your liver is clean and efficient, you will start to feel the subtle feedback your body communicates throughout the day. The itching after eating wheat, the constipation and/or loose bowel movements after eating out all weekend, the dull headaches after skipping breakfast and fueling up on coffee until noon. You'll have a comparative experience between feeling clear and energized and how you've gotten used to feeling when you don't make great choices about how you are fueling your body.

I know you would love me to give you an eating plan. I don't have one. If you *need* one then stick to the eating plan in the post-purification pamphlet. There are so many fertility diets available for free download online. I am more concerned about your ideas about eating. Food is medicine. Food is also poison. My general rules around food are based on moderation and balance. Healthy choices. If you are relatively healthy and you are making good choices 80 percent of the time, your 20 percent choices, more than likely, will not be catastrophic. It's all perspective.

Choices, Choices, Choices

Here are some ideas to consider when choosing foods. This period of your life is not about punishment or restrictions. It's about nourishing and healing, supporting and fertilizing. A balanced diet with as few preservatives and chemicals as possible – let's not muck up the liver. Lots of veggies. *Corn is not a vegetable.* It is the most GMO grain on the market. So please, if you did not know this, you know it now.

Think seasonal. Foods that are abundant during certain seasons are meant to be eaten during those seasons. Think of all the squash and pomegranates that are available during the fall and holiday season. Watermelon in the summer. It's all seasonal and perfect. Watermelon is cooling and diuretic. It helps us manage the heat of the summer. Pears in the late fall / early winter help nourish and moisten the lungs and dry coughs. The seasonality of food happens for a reason. Grains should be kept to a minimum. It can be a tough one for many people used to having rice as the focal point of their meal. Unfortunately, it's not great for long term insulin management. Think about good fats. Not trans fats, but good, healthy, unadulterated fats. Organic butter, avocado, salmon, whole organic milk. Watch your sugar intake. Watch the yogurts and the creamers. Moderation. Remember, this is not about denial and restriction – it's about looking at different foods and combinations to fertilize your system. Walnuts, almonds, and cashews. Great sources of fiber and protein. Eggs and organic beef, poultry, and wild healthy fish are a great resource for trace minerals and protein.

I'm trying to convey the concepts of moderation and balance. I know some of you will need a written plan. That's easy. Understanding and digesting the bigger process behind the plan is something you keep for your life. This is the underlying foundation of Chinese medicine. Balance and moderation. In western medicine, we might think of homeostasis. When our diets support this state, then we allow ourselves to be as fertile as possible, no matter where we are in our reproductive years.

Fertility is way more than the capacity to get pregnant and have a baby. Being in a fertile state transcends the physical into the emotional and into the spiritual. It is all connected and interrelated.

Have you heard the term that your gut is your second brain? Western medicine is just starting to run with this. Have you heard that leaky gut and inflammation has a direct effect on thinking, learning, and memory impairment? This is not new or shocking. How many times have you felt awful after a night out? How often do you feel foggy and fatigued after a cruise? We override our bodies' communication and suppress the symptoms. This works well until it doesn't.

A word about supplementation. Not all supplements are the same. Please know this is true. I am a board-certified herbalist. I am not a nutritionist. With that being said, food therapy is under my scope of practice as an acupuncture physician. It is, in fact, a foundation of Chinese medicine practice. Many patients never have acupuncture. Most take whole food nutritional supplements and alter their diets. They may also take Chinese herbal formulas.

What's in the Bag?

When they come in on their first visit, they show up with a bag of supplements. Sometimes they take pictures of all the vitamins because it's too much to carry! The supplements more often than not are poor quality and inefficient. They are loaded with fillers that need to be filtrated though the liver. It's the wild west out there! I have spent years educating myself about nutrition and products. Standard Process is my number one company for products. They are whole-food-based with the best clinical results. I have *never* been able to take vitamins without feeling nauseous and gaggy. I never felt better from anything I took and therefore could not be consistent. I went into my programs with tons of enthusiasm and high hopes. I always fell off the wagon because I couldn't digest the products, until I began using Standard Process products ten years ago. Not only do I see results on a daily basis in practice with patients, but when I skip my supplements for a handful of days, I really feel off.

Real Patient Story

Lauren came to us when she was 31 years old. She was a nurse and a newlywed. She was smart and great at taking care of everyone but herself. She knew she had PCOS, but she wasn't aware that she could help herself without prescription medications. She wanted to start getting regular periods so she could try to get pregnant. Lauren had been on the birth control pill for years in an effort to regulate her cycles. Without the birth control, she never had a period. She also took metformin to help her manage her borderline insulin resistance. She had had a whirlwind year planning her wedding, getting married, going on a honeymoon, and moving into a new home. Lots of celebration and new beginnings. She was exhausted, bloated, and fatigued. She was also emotionally volatile after coming off of the birth control after so many years. She knew she needed to get her health under control before she could even think about conceiving. Her gynecologist referred her to our office. She was 100 percent on board. Lauren was an ideal candidate for our 21-day liver purification. It made total sense to clear out the last year of party pollution from her liver. After she completed the purification, she continued with our post-purification recommendations and started taking some whole food nutrition products to regulate ovulation as well as nourish the integrity of her uterine lining. This is my fancy wording for infusing the uterus with nutrient dense blood flow. After four months of regular care, Lauren got her first natural period. It was a glimmer of light! Lauren discontinued her metformin because her fasting blood sugars were regulated. She treated with us for about a year when she found herself naturally pregnant. Due to her history of borderline insulin resistance, her doctors were concerned about gestational diabetes. She was monitored throughout her entire pregnancy. She would often say that she never felt better than she did while she was pregnant. She went on to deliver a beautiful baby boy. She recovered well, breastfed, and lost her baby weight like a healthy body is capable of doing.

PCOS patients can be a tough population to work with. We know that diet is critical to the success of managing PCOS. I actually introduced this 21-day liver purification program into my practice because of the growing PCOS populations. I needed to find a plan that was doable and practical. It's not only provided support and success for my PCOS patients but for all patients who could use a tune-up and reinvigoration of their health. This program has helped patients with endometriosis, multiple IVF cyclers, auto-immune patients, and basically every patient who is trying to enhance their bodies wisdom to say "*Yes.*"

Chapter Six

Timing is Everything

Timing is everything. We've heard this all of our lives. Whether you're a musician, an athlete, a photographer, or an accountant: right timing of sunlight, perfect timing of sequence, filing taxes on time, and being in the right place at the right time. Fertility and baby-making is not an exception to this phenomenon. In fact, timing is critical to the success of baby-making. How can you possibly capitalize on right timing? This is the question I will attempt to answer.

As a woman, there is a general awareness of timing in relationship to your menstrual cycle. If you are not connected to it, then its's close to impossible to learn the nuances that your body is trying to convey to you about your reproductive capacity. The rhythm of your cycle can and should be somewhat predictable. There are two sections of the cycle: the follicular phase and the luteal phase. The follicular phase begins on day one of your menstrual bleed. You are discharging your endometrial lining while your body is preparing to recruit antral follicles for the next round of ovulation. Once you ovulate, you enter into the luteal phase. The luteal phase should be 13 to 14 days. If you become pregnant, the cycle breaks and you do not revert back to a follicular phase. The rhythm of this process is elegant and meaningful. Hormones are secreted at certain intervals and the opportunity for fertilization and implantation exists within a designated window.

The great majority of women I treat have suppressed their normal monthly cycle for long periods of time. They have been on oral or injectable birth control to suppress their monthly bleed for a host of reasons. The most common reasons are due to underlying conditions that go untreated, like endometriosis, PCOS, heavy and painful cycles, and irregular cycling. Taking birth control might seem like a great solution to the immediate problem but in fact it does not treat the problem at all. It creates a "time out" from the symptoms that more often than not reappear when they discontinue the medication. This usually occurs when the woman is ready to start thinking about having a family and getting pregnant. It is way easier to resolve these underlying issues at a young age than it is when a woman is 36.

The healing and connection to your body's fertility rhythm is readily accessible. We all know we are having our period when we start bleeding! But how do you know when you are ovulating? How do you know *if* you are even ovulating? If you tend to have a 30-day cycle, the likelihood is that you are ovulating about mid-cycle. Start looking for signs starting around day 12 through day 16. It's not an exact science, as far as the day, but there will be subtle signs *if* you dial in. You may feel some extra activity in your lower abdomen. Some women feel slight cramping or discomfort around this time. You might have an increase in your libido. This is good! You might also have increased cervical discharge. These are all subtle signs that your body is on the verge of ovulation. When we have an awareness of our bodies' hormonal rhythm, then we can capitalize on the window of opportunity.

Menstrual cycling is influenced by many factors. I have patients who are night shift workers, pilots and flight attendants, international business executives, and full-time insomniacs! When your sleep cycle is dysfunctional, the rest of the body suffers. Sleep is extremely important for reproductive hormones. One of the foundational teachings in Chinese medicine is centered around the circadian rhythm of the body. Each system in the body has a two-hour window of optimal fullness and functionality. Beyond the actual 24-hour circadian rhythm of organ function, there is a seasonality to organ strength and weakness as well. One of the big differences between a holistic approach to health and healing is the inclusion of patterns and cycles in a patient's environment. In western medicine, the treatment is focused on diagnosis and disease. This is a generalization, but it is pretty accurate from what I see clinically. So how can cycles help improve your body's chance of saying yes? What is generally your best time of year? What is your worst time of the year? How are your sleep cycles? Do you have problems falling asleep? Staying asleep? Do you feel well rested when you wake up? All of these answers can reveal patterns specific to you and how you can improve your body's terrain to support conception and pregnancy.

Clean While You Sleep

Our bodies go through three consecutive two-hour cleaning cycles every night. The cycle can take fifteen minutes to two hours to initiate once we are laying horizontal. This means, for some people, that they need to be horizontal for eight hours in order for their systems to complete this cleansing cycle. I'm talking about liver, large intestine, small intestine, bladder and kidney, and every other cell and gland involved in cleansing the body. How many people do we all know that sleep for eight solid hours and wake up feeling fabulous? How many do you know that do not? When we correct sleep pattern with our fertility patients, we see hormonal irregularities rebalance.

The most common time that women wake up during sleep is between the hours of 1 and 3 a.m. This is the circadian window of the liver energy. The liver is responsible for the smooth and sequential flow of qi and blood in the body. When the liver energy is not flowing well, we use the term "liver qi stagnation." This can give rise to frustration, angst, irritability, and other lovely emotional states. Waking within this one to three am window is a clue to an imbalanced liver meridian. The liver meridian courses through the reproductive organs, so it is essential for the liver system to be open, flowing, and balanced.

Most medical doctors will not discuss sleep or menstrual cycling with a patient in great detail. I will. It is also important to understand the patterns and seasons of how your body soars and struggles. Most patients have a time of year that they are run down and susceptible to asthma, headaches, allergies, eczema flare-ups, or bronchitis, etc....

This speaks to the person's underlying weakness. All of the small signs and symptoms in relations to the time of day, the season, or the year paint a picture of a patient's overall health. This picture can help support how to reestablish a healthy rhythm to the body and that in turn can increase a patient's natural capacity to conceive.

The point here is that the disconnection from your body, your environment, and your patterns of health can lead you further away from your natural capacity to conceive. My suggestion is to reconnect and get back to the basics. If you are lost as to where you can begin, I would recommend with sunrise and sunset. The sun slowly rises and ascends. It peaks by noon. From noon on, it slowly descends and finally sets. This cycle happens day in and day out, year after year. It works. What I tend to see is that people get up and want to be *up*. They are fueled with caffeine and then around 10 – 10:30 a.m., they are looking for another bump to stay *up* until lunchtime. I then see the habit of the bump *up* reoccur around 2 – 2:30 in the afternoon. I refer to these two slump periods of the day as the Starbucks, Coke, Red Bull, Dunkin Donuts power hours! These slump periods are followed by the 10 – 11p.m. Benadryl, Tylenol PM, Ambien, Lunesta hour! It's getting late, you're still wired up, and you have to be up at 6:45 a.m. so you need to get to sleep! This is considered normal for many people. Long term, this routine will wreak havoc on your health and completely contribute to hormonal imbalance.

Real Patient Story

Jennifer came to our office to help her get her weight and PCOS symptoms under control. She was 27 years old, obese, and being medicated for insulin resistance and high blood pressure. She was a pharmacist. She worked seven days on and seven days off. She chose to work this shift because it paid a substantial amount more than a regular schedule and she wanted to make enough money to pay off her student loans in three years. She had been working this shift for the past year and had gained 30 pounds. She was overweight to begin with, so the extra 30 pounds compounded her health problems. When she was working her seven-day shift, she was able to catch catnaps here and there, but she never had long periods of restful sleep. She also ate all of her meals at the hospital because the pharmacy she worked at was in the hospital. I had her journal her food and drink choices along with all the snacks, cokes, and coffees over a week's shift. When she kept track of what she was eating and drinking, she was shocked at how much garbage she ate and drank. I am telling you, the lifestyle journals are very eye-opening. It also became clear that Jennifer was rarely sleeping more than two hours at any period of time when she was working her seven-day shift. She never got close to a full horizontal cleansing cycle in any seven-day work shift. When we really examined her lifestyle, it was clear that for half of the month, she was creating a toxic cycle of poor sleep, poor nutrition, and chronic elevated blood sugars.

The obvious solution would begin with Jennifer changing her work schedule. She was not open to making that change for at least another year. The financial stress of her student loans was the worse of two evils compared to her unhealthy work schedule. We created a selection of food choices and drink options to help keep her nourished and hydrated during her seven-day work week. She started taking adrenal and sugar-regulating supplements that made her cravings and energy levels more balanced. She was able to shop the week she had off to fill in her food choices with healthier options. She worked out a sleep schedule with another pharmacist that they did their best to adhere to. The night shift was not as demanding as the early morning and mid-day requirements. When Jennifer got four to six hours of uninterrupted sleep, she felt significantly better. Jennifer had regular acupuncture treatments when she was off from work. Over a six-month period, she lost 26 pounds and was able to reduce her medications.

Jennifer has been under care for the past 18 months. She continues to lose weight and restore her hormonal system. She has started having regular menstrual cycles and positive ovulation tests. It has been a long road, but as she has changed her lifestyle, her health has improved. She has just been approved for a normal 40-hour week schedule. I am confident as she continues to improve her sleep habits and lifestyle choices, she will restore healthy reproductive function.

Right timing transcends all living processes. Is anyone really an overnight success? Isn't it all possible that the timing is always right and we could be imposing our expectations and plans on the right timing for our child to come through? I think about this and many other philosophically-minded ideas on a daily basis. I see miracles happen all the time. I am convinced that babies come exactly when they are meant to. They come through when all odds are against you and they come through when all the doctors, tests, and procedures conclude that it won't happen. My best strategy for all patients is to get them as healthy as possible so the body can say yes. I know it sounds hokey and unscientific and like new age positive thinking blah blah blah, but if you see results pointing to one common factor, it's impossible to ignore it.

Another thought to leave you with. How is it that when a couple finally gives up, surrenders, and moves on do they find themselves pregnant? I have so many stories that end up like this. I have friends who have two children ages 13 and 11. They were both conceived though IVF. They were told that they would *never* conceive without IVF. Three years ago, my friend, 42 years old, found herself naturally pregnant. She now has a two-and-a-half-year-old healthy baby boy. Her husband was furious and enraged. He wanted all his money back from the IVF clinic that he spent 14 years ago! How does this all happen? Right timing, trust, and intimate relations!

Chapter Seven

You Are Not Your Labs

L ab results are a Kodak moment in time. Labs are not a final determination of your health. Too many patients decide certain things about themselves based on their labs. IVF clinics and many practitioners add fuel to the fire by labeling a patient's condition with a diagnosis. Then, you, the patient, believe with all your heart that you have "old eggs," "you're a Clomid failure" or that your egg quality is poor. If you are close to 35 years old, you will be further pressured by the biological ticking time bomb. I invite you to *pause*. Lab values are information. The important thing to remember is that the body is a vital intricate orchestration that is able to improve, heal, and self-correct. It is very rare that a patient cannot improve their health. The healthier you are, the greater likelihood that your body will say yes to pregnancy.

I have been working in the infertility arena for 20 years. The science of reproductive endocrinology is relatively young. The oldest IVF baby at the time of this writing is on the verge of turning 40. Louise Brown was conceived through IVF because her mother did not have fallopian tubes. This procedure was created to help a woman conceive because she had a structural problem. Today IVF is used for many other reasons. It's a life-changing process for patients that really need it. It can be a nightmare for many others who try to override their problems with the hopes of IVF being a "magic elixir." It is not a magic wand that overcomes unhealthy function. Remember that getting and staying pregnant will always be a stress event on the body. The body will always self-protect and prioritize how it uses its resources. Often not getting or staying pregnant is an attempt to keep you in the game of your life.

Years ago, the lab values for fertility assessment were dominated by a few numbers. A patient's fertility prognosis was determined by their day 3 FSH (follicle stimulating hormone) and E2 (estradiol), their antral follicle count, and their age. These were the "big four" My first successes with patients were those patients that were convinced that they were not going to be mothers because they had high

FSH. This was a prison sentence and a state of mind that women were walking around with. We had great success with this population. When patients were retested after working with our practice over a three- to four-month period, their labs improved substantially. I began to see how valuable diet, sleep, high quality nutritional products, herbs, and mental state were in influencing the body's capacity to heal and say yes to fertility.

One of the newer and heavily respected lab values that play into the prognosis of fertility is a woman's AMH. AMH stands for anti-Mullerian hormone. AMH is secreted by the immature granulosa cells of the ovarian follicles. This lab value can be tested on any day of the menstrual cycle. Low AMH levels are equated to poor egg reserve. High AMH levels can relate to PCOS. Again, we must remember that this value can change and only represents a moment in time when the labs were drawn. AMH seems to have trumped all other labs. Fertility clinics love to tell patients that their reserves are dwindling and that the sooner you do an IVF the better your chances are of getting pregnant. This further contributes to your desperation and bad decision-making. Making decisions from this mental state is never a good strategy.

Great Docs Are Out There!

Fortunately, there are some great physicians out there that understand the value of healthy lifestyle changes and the impact that they can have on your fertility outcomes. First of all, it's important to look at your whole body to make a good assessment regarding your fertility potential. We like to look at fasting blood sugar levels, cholesterol levels, homocysteine levels, thyroid function in addition to all the standard fertility markers. This is a whole-body orchestration. When I see elevated inflammation markers, then I already know that the body is trying to reduce inflammation and self-protect. No organ or gland operates in a vacuum. The woodwinds work in harmony with the strings and the percussion sections – it's not a solo performance. When we reduce inflammation and move body fat levels out of obesity range, we see lab values change and fertility enhanced. It's not some special sauce that we are selling. It's common sense, moderation, and small consistent changes that improve your health.

Yes, This Can Happen for You

One of the main reasons I am writing this book is to let you know that you are not your labs. You do not have to be that desperate and hopeless woman who thinks that her ship has sailed. I can say for sure that 75 percent of the cases that I see that are diagnosed "old eggs" and "poor reserve" go on to have healthy children. When you consult with a reproductive endocrinologist, they are hearing you say that you want a baby and you want it now. You have been trying and have not been successful. Fast tracking your process with IVF is not a slam dunk. IVF is the main process that a reproductive endocrinologist has to offer. Don't be upset or blame yourself that that you have landed here. This is what they do. You are actually *not* a good candidate for IVF with high FSH and low AMH levels. Why? The medications that are used in IVF to stimulate more follicles do not work well when these numbers are not in a certain range. It's not that you cannot get pregnant – it's that you will not respond well to their process. But if you are desperate enough you might be willing to go through the process because there is a 30 percent chance that you might override the natural process. The ticking biological clock is always a pressure push that further supports a "hurry-up-and-fail" game plan. I am not saying that IVF cycles always fail; I am saying that getting as healthy as possible before a cycle will always be your best strategy for success.

Typically, women from 39 to 45 will have low AMH. Their antral follicle counts will be on the low side as well.

Their chances for success are far lower with IVF than a younger woman's. These are great candidates for natural conception. The exception to all of this is when a woman has blocked or damaged fallopian tubes. This is a structural issue that is best served by IVF like it was originally intended over 40 years ago. But a woman who has a less than 5 percent chance of success with IVF is our favorite population to work with. Generally speaking, most IVF clinics will recommend donor egg IVF to this patient. This is a $30,000 process that does not come with a 75 percent success rate outcome. Most women are willing to try getting healthy and conceiving naturally first.

Real Patient Story

Sharon had been trying to conceive for over three years. She got married at 41 and knew her odds were not great. She decided to get evaluated with an IVF doctor. He told her that her chances were less than 2% with IVF. Not only was her egg reserve and quality diminished, but her husband had some sperm issues. She decided she had nothing to lose by getting healthy. She was 44 when she began working with my office. We evaluated her lifestyle assessment journals and had her start making changes immediately. She changed her diet and exercise regime and started taking high quality nutritional supplements. Although we weren't treating her for her acne or her thinning hair and inability to lose weight, she started to see all of these improve over the first three months of treatment. She also noticed that her signs of ovulation were stronger: cervical discharge and an increase in her libido! Her husband started taking high quality nutritional sperm support and he too noticed an overall improvement in how he was feeling. We were not retesting any labs or sending her for ultrasounds. It took close to a year for Sharon to become pregnant. She was 45 years old now so she was definitely considered a high-risk pregnancy. She had some early testing in the first trimester that indicated her pregnancy was healthy and normal. Sharon went on to deliver a gorgeous, healthy, Buddha baby. I say Buddha baby because this little girl was the most robust, alert baby I had seen in years. All the babies that come through our practice are beautiful and miraculous in my eyes, but Sharon's baby girl was exceptional.

Sharon spent less than $5000.00 in my practice over an 18-month period. She conceived at 45 and delivered at 46. Going into her pregnancy, she was probably healthier than she had been in the past ten years of her life. She continued to maintain her healthy lifestyle post-partum so she could breast-feed her daughter. I will admit that I was thrilled beyond belief to witness her process. I have had many patients after her that followed in her footsteps, but she still holds the record for being the oldest patient to naturally conceive and deliver in my practice.

Additional Patient Story

Laurie came to our office when she was 30. She came to get help with regulating her cycles and she also needed help recognizing when and if she was ovulating. She had been on the birth control pill for the past ten years. Her gynecologist put her on the pill to help regulate her cycle. Now that she was married, she wanted to come off birth control. She wanted to give her body a chance to regulate and prepare herself for the possibility of getting pregnant. It took four months of regular herbs and acupuncture before Laurie got her first menstrual cycle. She had one more cycle 35 days later. She continued with treatment and didn't get another cycle for over two months. She decided she should consult with a specialist while working with our practice. Her labs indicated that she had POF (premature ovarian failure). She had undetectable AMH and a very low antral follicle count. She was devastated. The reproductive endocrinologist highly recommended doing a few cycles of stimulation to batch her embryos.

She decided that she was too stressed out to make a move, so she continued treating in our office until she was ready. Four months later, Laurie became naturally pregnant. She miscarried at seven weeks. The entire pregnancy was so improbable with her history. She was encouraged, though. She *never* had a regular period until she came under care in our practice, so she was willing to continue with treatment and see how her body would respond. She became pregnant again after three months. At the time of this writing, she is 22 weeks pregnant. She is well into her second trimester and all tests indicate that she is carrying a healthy baby.

I can't tell you how many women come into my office committed to their lab values and diagnosis. This can mentally and emotionally cripple a patient and influence every waking moment of her day. She will look for proof and evidence on the internet to put nails in her fertility coffin, almost like she is building a case against herself and her potential to conceive. All I can say is that most of the time, it's just not true. If your current labs indicate a poor prognosis for fertility, then you have options. You are not stuck in that lab value. The body is vital, dynamic, and resilient. Give yourself a chance to restore balance and optimal hormonal function. When you make committed lifestyle changes and nourish yourself with high-grade supplements and healthy food choices, you have an opportunity to rewrite your story.

Chapter Eight

Staying the Course, Overcoming Obstacles, and Exploring Options

Ugh … sometimes it seems like this is never going to happen. I know how this feels. I too didn't understand why it was all so difficult to just have a baby, adopt a baby, afford a baby, etc. People have been doing it since the beginning of time. *Why is it so hard for me?* Sometimes there are no real answers and sometimes there are some plausible answers. Regardless, it can still be a grind. In the end, when you do become a parent, you will more than likely forget how desperate and difficult your darkest moments were.

I know patients who have spent years trying to create a family. It can suck the life out of you. Beyond the emotional strife, it really can impact your physical health. I am sure if you are reading this, then you know the financial burden all these high-tech procedures and meds can create. This is something I have spent my entire career trying to help patients avoid and mitigate. Unless you have a structural issue, like blocked tubes for example or no egg reserve at all (rare, but I have seen this), please consider taking a deep breath and a momentary pause. I am not saying stop... just pause to get some clarity and perspective.

Over the past 20 years, it has become more common place for a woman to think, "I just figured I would do IVF when I was ready to have a baby." This was one of the last options a woman ever considered when I first began working with fertility patients. Now it's as commonplace as owning a cell phone. Additionally, women have the option of freezing their eggs and putting their baby-making on ice for an indefinite period of time. Egg freezing is different than embryo freezing because it doesn't require sperm ... meaning a husband, significant other, or donor! Many progressive corporations like Google and Apple offer financial assistance for their employees so they don't feel the pressure of the biological clock during their most fertile years.

You Do Have Options

Know that there are always options. In Chapter Four, we went into detail about your head game. It is pretty overwhelming to think and believe that you do not have options. In fact, we are living in a remarkable time in reproductive medicine. I am not saying that this is your *first* thought or option, but assisted reproductive therapies offer life-changing options for many couples. I will repeat my mantra though: Getting as healthy as possible before doing any assisted reproductive therapy is always your best strategy.

There is always the option to adopt. Again, for most people this is generally not the first thought a couple has. Adoption is not a slam dunk process either. It's not like you go into a store and pick out a baby. The process is rigorous and detailed and it's designed that way in an effort to protect and ensure that a child is being given to a good family. I know many couples that have fostered to adopt with no financial cost and I know families that have spent large sums of money to adopt. I have patients that have naturally conceived children and also adopted children into their family. The point is there is no right way, good way, perfect way, or promised way. Families are created in unlimited ways today, like never before. The more attached you are to "how it has to be," the more likely you will struggle. This is real life and more times than not, it tends to unfold with a lot of twists and turns that you could never foresee. Always know that when you think there are no options that your lens is ready to be widened and expanded if you have the courage to do so.

It's Always and Never the Right Time!

Believe it or not, this is perfect training for being a parent. There will be so many days and nights that tend to bleed into each other where you will wonder how you will ever get through this "period." The first year of your child's life, with little to no sleep, will be one of them. Eighteen months through three years old, riddled with tantrums, toilet training, and complete exhaustion from the boundless toddler energy and curiosity will be another. Every parent gets through it. Even with zero experience. Even when they've read every book and it's useless information in the moment your kid is screaming bloody murder in the middle of your local grocery store! Not having things go as you planned is 100 percent guaranteed when you are a parent. The pre-parent phase is starting earlier for you. This is your fertility process and it doesn't have to be a nightmare.

On average, most patients spend about two years working with me. They conceive in a variety of ways. One way or another, families get created. I work with patients through preconception, pregnancy, delivery, and post-partum care. More often than not, I see them within a few years to have baby number two. If a patient goes on to adoption, I help guide them through that process as well. My goal is to get all patients closer to their family.

I am a team player and our practice works with many supportive practitioners. It would be unrealistic to think that I could provide everything for every patient. Sometimes I am the absolutely wrong person to be working with. I will happily refer a patient to a "good fit" for them. This is about you and your dream and I have learned to not take any of this personally and be of service to you whether or not I can personally help you. If you, for any reason, feel that you are not being heard or respected by your practitioners, I implore you to make a move. Having a baby and creating a family is the most important thing you will ever do. More important than buying a home, getting married, or writing a book! Your child is your child forever. You do not ever need to endure dismissive, arrogant, non-compassionate care when you are seeking medical help. This is unacceptable and as a patient advocate, I will always try to guide you to like-minded, respectful practitioners.

Another word of advice is to reread Chapter Four. If you feel like you are being rushed into a procedure – and that you are being shuffled into a fast decision – you probably are. I am not saying that all IVF clinics operate like this. There are many that are amazing and highly ethical and leaders in the science and business of assisted reproductive therapy. Then there are those that are not. Always trust your instinct and gut feeling.

Staying the Course

I'm going to list a bunch of options that patients have investigated, explored, and experienced. Trust me, they were not, in most cases, their first choice:

Clomid. Clomid with timed intercourse. Clomid with IUI. Injectable meds with IUI. IVF. IVF with ICSI. Batching embryos through multiple IVF cycles. Frozen embryo transfer. IVF with PGS. Donor egg IVF. Donor Sperm with IVF. IVF with surrogacy. Donor egg with surrogacy. Foster to adopt. Adoption. Giving up. Getting pregnant naturally.

I'm not a statistical genius, not even close, but these are just a few of the common ways patients create their families. Interestingly, I have many patients who go through the entire marathon and, as I shared earlier in the book, they end up becoming pregnant naturally after the marathon is over. So, when you think you are out of options, I would venture to say you probably are not even close.

Marathon Mentality

Staying the course. I want you to know why this area of medicine chose me. Let me say it was a mutual choice in that I also chose fertility. Happily. There will never be a patient more committed than a fertility patient. I understand the bigger vision and desire to want something so badly that you are willing to do whatever it takes to have it happen. *No matter what.* I felt that way about my life disrupting endometriosis. I had so much to do in my life that I felt driven to any limit to resolve my problem. *No matter what.* Fertility patients have a similar drive and vision. Having a baby is a base, guttural longing that every woman believes is her right. It tends to hit us stronger and louder at different times in our life. We can't ignore it. It's part of our fabric, our cells, and our deep feminine core. It is almost unexplainable because it is so deeply felt. When a patient is driven by this longing she will be compliant, committed, and, more often than not, successful. My caution is to watch the ledge of desire as it neighbors on the edge of desperation and loss of perspective. This neighborhood can lead us to bad decision making and unhealthy choices. This is where the circus and the roller coaster consume your every waking moment. They even disrupt your sleep. This is when you get to pause and reconnect with your instinct and vision. This is a marathon, not a sprint. When you run a marathon like a sprinter, you will never finish.

When something you want so badly keeps evading you, it can wear you down emotionally and spiritually. I often recommend that patients journal or speak to a therapist that specializes in fertility. This journey can be very isolating and lonely. There are nonprofit groups that meet in an effort to hold space for this journey. They are not for everyone. Sometimes it can turn into a complaint session and it can be very scary for patients who are just beginning to navigate fertility options. Sometimes it can be lifesaving. Each group has its own vibe. If you feel inclined, try it out. In our practice, we have an informal fertility buddy process. If a patient expresses a desire to connect with another like-minded patient, we make connections for them – of course, with both parties' consent. I have patients who have become best friends over the years because of these introductions. They are raising their kids together and share a period of time that was once overwhelming and hopeless. These origins of friendship are replaced by child rearing challenges and joys. This is the real marathon.

The Power of Your Words

I want you to notice throughout this book I rarely use the term infertility. Whether or not you know the true definition of infertility, it implies that you cannot have a baby. I hate it. It's a spiritual downer and I refuse to use it. I have rarely met an infertile patient. I have worked with over a thousand patients that were in a sub-fertile state. My treatment is always to improve fertility and overall health so the body will be more likely to say yes to pregnancy. Be careful with your language. It is very powerful. The constant thought that "I am infertile and my eggs are old" does not serve your higher self. There is nothing empowering or inspiring about this conversation. It is also in most cases not 100 percent true.

When you reach the point of giving up and throwing in the towel, know that you are on the verge of breaking through. I have repeatedly seen patients take a break and give up "for now." Sometimes it's a good idea. It's also a good idea to get a second opinion and try something different. I have seen patients stick with a clinic for multiple cycles of failed procedures. When they switch doctors or clinics and try a different protocol, they seem to have miraculous success. Is it really a miracle? I think all babies that make their way through are miracles, and these cases are no different. It just appears to the patient in their experience that this outcome is miraculous. Hang on to that possibility because realistically, these outcomes happen all the time.

Chapter Nine

Conclusion

Thank you for coming on this journey with me. As I wrote the book, I have had the opportunity to think about the hundreds and probably thousands of patients that I've treated. That alone was worth the courage, time, and energy I have had to access to share this with you. You are just as likely to have a great and inspiring result with the Fertility Fuel process. I have written this book for you. I am oftentimes outraged and saddened by the negative information that is shared with the masses. It's not the full story. I have had the honor and good fortune to help so many women and couples call forth a life. Their baby. One way or another they broke through. This is my wish for you.

In the introduction and the first few chapters, I let you know that I know who you are. I have worked with you and I get it. I was on the same quest. My details were different but the longing was the same. Our issues are not so "special and unique." We of course love to think that they are but, in fact, human beings have been wanting the same things forever. We happen to be living in a time of great distraction and disconnection but we are still human beings. We want love, connection, family, and acceptance. When the cell phone, laptop, TV, and headphones are all turned off, we are left with ourselves, our spouses, friends, family, and coworkers. We crave connection beyond Facebook likes. The ultimate connection is that of a parent to a child.

I know you deeply understand the miracle that you are trying to create. Yes, so much more than the sperm and the egg. You know that even when everything is "perfect" and all the labs point to "unexplained" that you are in fact asking for a miracle. You know that when you bypass the obstacles with high tech science and it still doesn't work that you are praying for a miracle. You especially know that each time you lost a pregnancy that when you are down on your knees praying, you are asking for a miracle to come through. This is what we are up to.

When you have reached your tipping point, your point of surrender, your last straw, and your rope's end, you will happily widen your lens and see the bigger picture that was always there. There is hope and there are options. I promise.

I shared how my son came to me. I had been dreaming about him most of my life. I never expected it to be so difficult and then so easy. It was on his time. Not mine. When he was ready, it was easy. Five consecutive days of grace. It was so hard to trust this. The more I imposed my schedule, my timing, and my stuff onto the process, the more difficult life became – all aspects of my life. It spilled into my marriage, my joy, my work, and my health. When I let go and got back to everything else that I had created up until that point, the river became less turbulent. Things started flowing again. Learning to pick up on the nuances of your life can help steer you into the right places and situations. I see how this happens for myself and for patients all the time. I am not special. What I am is tuned in and connected.

When you work with me, I will listen to your story. The whole story. All the uncomfortable details. The frustration and the sadness. The guilt and the shame. You are free to lay it all out. When you allow yourself to flush it out, you create a space for something different. You may also realize that some of that story is just not true. If you need to be angry, sad, or quiet for a while, then you get to do that too. At some point, you will reconnect with your bigger vision of creating a family and you will be ready to make a move.

Midway through *Fertility Fuel* you discovered that all the small choices that you make on a daily basis are way more important than you ever thought. You got to really look at the breakdown of the details. For example, you can see how if you consume two teaspoons of sugar in two cups of coffee every day, seven days a week, this adds up to 28 teaspoons a week. 52 multiplied by 28 equals 1,456 teaspoons of sugar. *This is over thirteen pounds of sugar* without even eating anything that contains sugar, fructose, sucrose, etc. It's the unconscious automatic pilot choices that make the difference. This of course is a common example, but the point is you have the opportunity to make small changes, compounded daily, that can enhance your capacity to conceive.

You will have an opportunity to connect with your intuition. Your inner guide and inner knowing will be waiting. There will be a big "welcome-back-home" hug. It will be a rekindling of the safest, wisest place on the planet. This is where you will gather strength and learn to rebuild trust in what you already possess.

I shared the importance of right timing, and the necessity of living in harmony with the circadian rhythm that has been ruling the cycles of nature from the beginning of time. Learning to adjust and acclimate to the cycle of the sunrise, high noon, and sunset, the moon cycles, and the cycle of the seasons will accelerate your body's innate timing. Hormonal release, ovulation, sleep, energy highs and lows, and mood balance all connect to these cycles.

Following my discussion on timing was the chapter on lab values. So many of us create an identity about ourselves based on our lab values. "I am PCOS. I have old eggs. I do not ovulate and I have to do IVF. I can't get pregnant because I have a fatty liver and I'm a Clomid failure." All too often, a single round of labs is drawn, conclusions are made, and medications are prescribed to alter the labs. I am not against medications when they are necessary. I do believe that changing daily habits and modifying lifestyle can in many instances change the labs and the overall health and fertility potential of the majority of patients *without* negative side effects. Oh yes, there will be side effects of the changes I prescribe. Big time. The most common side effects will be weight loss, stable blood sugars, improved sleep, regular ovulation, reduction in moodiness, increased libido and joy, and overall enhancement of fertility potential. Labs need to be looked at for patterns. The ovaries don't operate autonomously. They are a part of a hormonal symphony. Listening to the full piece of music often reveals the weak links and patterns of imbalance.

Keeping your head and heart in the game is the last chapter of the process. It's a marathon. Even after you have your child, you will realize that you are just beginning! You may have sought counsel from various doctors, specialists, coaches, and support blogs up until this point. It hasn't worked. Now you are here. Now you have read this book and maybe something changed for you and maybe you know what your next step is. Maybe you have the clarity to make the changes and get your head in the right space to make better choices to have your dream come to fruition. I am thrilled and 100 percent your biggest fan and wish you all the joy and fulfillment I know a child can offer. If anything that you read in this book moved you in a forward direction or touched your heart in some small way, I have accomplished my purpose.

If you still feel that you could use some support and detailed methodology to help move you in the direction of your dreams coming true, you have an opportunity to work with me directly. This is what I do. You would think that after doing this for so many years that it would become stale and routine. *Never*. When a person discovers their inherent gift, it is useless unless it is shared. This is my gift.

I am really good at connecting with the miracle that you are and the one that you are trying to call forth. I do not work with everyone. I work with women who are ready to break through the stories, bad doctoring, and Dr. Google confusion. You do not have to fly to my office to see me. My program is virtual and it is one-on-one with me at this point in time. I have relationships with great practitioners all over the United States, Europe, and Canada if you need to be referred out for tests and local acupuncture. Fertility Fuel is a 90-day program that has the potential to change your life. If you are fed up, overwhelmed, and discouraged by your current treatment or prognosis, it is probably the perfect time to fill your tank with Fertility Fuel. If you are just starting out and want to get as healthy as possible to improve your chances of creating a family, Fertility Fuel can be the perfect place to begin.

In closing, I want to let you know that it is my greatest pleasure and honor to be a part of your process. Allowing me to help you in any way create the space for a child to come through is my zone of genius and my life's work. I have wanted to efficiently and effectively help more women for years beyond the geography of my beautiful office in Delray Beach, FL. If you feel compelled to have my support through this process, you can fill out a request for a free fifteen-minute discovery call and you will be contacted to schedule an appointment.

About the Author

Susan G. Schiff, DOM, is a nationally board-certified Acupuncture Physician and herbalist. She is a diplomate fellow of the American Board of Oriental Reproductive Medicine. She is one of the original Fertile Soul practitioners mentored by Dr. Randine Lewis. She has helped 100s of couples create families over the past 20 years in her Palm Beach county office. Dr. Schiff collaborates with some of the top reproductive endocrinology doctors, locally and virtually.

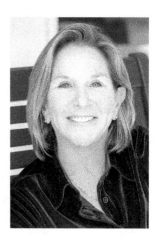

Dr. Schiff was a patient before she became a practitioner. After years of palliative care with western medicine, she sought a deeper course of treatment to address the underlying dysfunction of her reproductive system. Chinese medicine changed her life and her life path. She chose to study the medicine that healed her. She has never looked back.

Dr. Schiff has studied with Chinese medicine masters in the United States, Canada, and China. She has done clinical hours in IVF clinics and embryology labs. Her zone of genius lies in her ability to integrate current day modern diagnosis and translate it into classic Chinese medicine treatment protocols.

If she is not in her clinic or traveling for education, Dr. Schiff can be found working on her golf game. She loves to explore the world with her family. She has been to South Africa, India, China, Europe, Dominican Republic, Bali, Thailand, Banff, Jasper, Vancouver, and all over the United States.

She lives in Delray Beach, Florida with her wife of 21 years, her 11-year-old son, and their two terriers.

Thank You

Thank you for spending your time reading *Fertility Fuel* and getting to know me and the Fertility Fuel program.

I am on a mission to restore hope and empower women and couples while they embark on one of the most unexpected and important journeys in their lives.

If you are looking for further support and guidance in creating your family, I am available to work with you. This program is virtual and available anywhere there is an internet connection.

Please send an email to discoverycall@FertilityFuel.com to set up a complimentary 15-minute call to see if you are a good fit for our program.

One last thought. Never forget that every life is a miracle. When you connect with the miracle that you are, you create the opening for another.